I QUIT

Cigarettes, Candy Bars & Booze

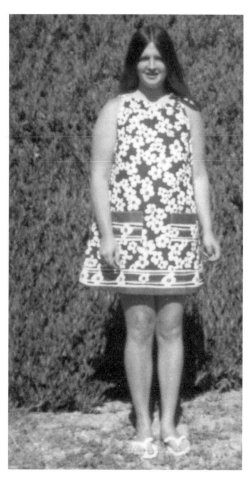

Linda at sixteen

As a teenager Linda Joy Allan weighed over two hundred pounds. When she was sixteen Linda smoked her first cigarette and didn't stop smoking for twenty-eight years. For twelve years she drank so heavily that she alienated most of her friends and family.

There were times when Linda felt so helplessly trapped in the grip of her addictions that she couldn't imagine overcoming any one of them, BUT SHE DID.

A true story, told with honesty and wit, reminding us of the power of human determination and self-preservation.

I QUIT

Cigarettes, Candy Bars & Booze

Linda Joy Allan

I QUIT
Cigarettes, Candy Bars & Booze

Published by Dovelin Publishing
3905 State Street, Suite 7-184
Santa Barbara, CA 93105-5107
www.dovelinpublishing.com
info@dovelinpublishing.com

Copyright © 2008 by Linda Joy Allan

Publisher's Cataloging-in-Publication

Allan, Linda Joy.

I quit : cigarettes, candy bars & booze / Linda Joy Allan. -- 1st ed. --
Santa Barbara, CA : Dovelin Publishing, 2008.

p. ; cm.
ISBN: 978-0-9779149-0-6 ; 0-9779149-0-9

1. Allan, Linda Joy--Substance abuse. 2. Allan, Linda Joy--
Biography. 3. Recovering addicts--Biography. 4. Recovering
alcoholics--Biography. 5. Substance abuse. 6. Compulsive eating.
7. Habit breaking. 8. Motivation (Psychology) 9. Self-realization.
10. Spirituality. I. Title.

BL625.9.R43 A45 2007   2006903786
248.8/629--dc22   0609

This publication is designed to educate and provide general information regarding
the subject matter covered. It is not intended to replace the counsel of other professional advisors. The reader is encouraged to consult with his or her own advisors
regarding specific situations. While the author has taken reasonable precautions in
the preparation of this book and believes the facts presented within the book are
accurate, neither the publisher nor the author assumes any responsibility for errors or
omissions. The publisher and author specifically disclaim any liability resulting from
the use or application of the information contained in this book. The information
within this book is not intended to serve as emotional or therapeutic advice related
to individual situations.

First Edition

Book Design: Robert Aulicino
Editor: Gail M. Kearns

Printed and bound in the United States of America on acid-free paper

This book is dedicated to
all those struggling with addiction

Contents

Acknowledgments

I want to thank everyone who cheered me on as this book was coming to fruition.

To my family, who thought the idea of my book was a great idea from the beginning. Thanks for all your input and support.

To my brother David — you left all too soon but your impact on my life will never be forgotten.

To Rita, Lori, Mary, Sharon and Margaret, whose constant encouragement helped me more than you know.

To my dear friend Allan — I never got tired of all the times you asked me, "What's new with the book?"

Introduction

EVERY DAY WE HEAR STORIES ABOUT PEOPLE STRUGGLING to overcome addictions. Famous movie stars pay tens of thousands of dollars to check themselves into rehab clinics to give up drinking. They come out clean and sober, but a few years later, they're right back in again. The ones who do succeed still identify themselves as alcoholics, because the struggle's never over.

For some people, compulsive eating is the addiction. They try every diet that comes out; they lose a little weight, then gain it all back again. It's frustrating, but they keep on trying, year after year, because nobody wants to be fat.

Cigarette smoking can be even worse. Almost forty-six million people in the United States are smokers. A lot of those people are trying to quit. They've tried nicotine patches, filter tips and cold turkey, but nothing seems to work.

In all the stories we hear, it sounds like not many people really win completely. Sooner or later, they always go back to their addictions. There are temporary victories, but very few permanent success stories. So we get the impression that it can't be done. But it can be done.

That's why I want to tell you my story. I want to let you know that someone out there has done it. I overcame all three of these addictions — drinking, compulsive eating and smoking.

At one point, I weighed over two hundred pounds, but I haven't eaten compulsively for over thirty years. According to the charts, I'm at my ideal weight.

For twelve years, I drank so heavily that I alienated my friends and family. I couldn't always remember where I'd parked my car or whom I'd slept with the night before. I lost one boyfriend after another because I wouldn't quit drinking. But I stopped drinking for good in 1987.

When I was sixteen, I smoked my first cigarette and I never stopped till I was forty-four. Smoking was the longest addiction. For twenty-eight years, smoking truly was like having a friend anytime I wanted it.

When I was sad, I reached for a cigarette. When I was happy, a cigarette could only add to my happiness. In a crowd of people, I was glad to have my cigarette along. When I was by myself — just my cigarette and me — it made my time alone more special. I looked forward to each one.

A cigarette is not fattening or intoxicating. It gives you a handy reason to take breaks throughout the day. Whether you're at work or at home in the middle of a project, you can look forward to taking a break every so often to have a cigarette. Then you're ready to get back to whatever you're doing.

I used to watch people like my mother, who never smoked a day in her life, and wonder, "How can they enjoy life without smoking?"

There were times when I felt so trapped in the grip of my addictions that I couldn't imagine overcoming any one of them. I tried to get to the root of the problem. I thought, If I can just understand why I'm so addicted to these things, I'll be able to stop.

Eventually, I realized that it didn't matter why. Maybe I'd find out one day, maybe I wouldn't. But, in the meantime, I just had to quit!

This is my story. I can't let you in on any secrets or make you any promises. All I can do is tell you what happened to me.

I can say with absolute certainty that it is possible to

give up an addiction, once and for all. I'm a living testament to that. And what I discovered is this: Once you quit, the struggling is over.

I don't go to parties and wish I could have a drink. I really don't want one any more. And once I decided to quit, there was no struggle. I just quit. The real struggle was living my life as an alcoholic, trying to make excuses for why things were falling apart, lying to myself and to the people I loved. Compared to that, quitting was easy.

The same is true for smoking or eating compulsively. My life would be nothing like it is now if I still had to live in a struggle with those addictions. I know I'll never go back to any one of them again.

Why would I ever trade this freedom for a cigarette or candy bar or booze?

1

Braveheart

HOSPITALS ARE SO LONELY. MY MOST VIVID MEMORIES OF being four and five years old take place in hospitals. Even today, if I step into the long, empty corridors of a hospital that reeks with illness and that antiseptic smell, I can see myself lying alone, night after night, behind the bars of a crib, crying silently.

I mainly missed my mom on those nights. She had such a gentle voice and tender way about her. The hospital was the antithesis of loving care. Impersonal, sterile, not concerned about comforting a lonely child, it was stark and filled with unpleasantness for me.

The nurses in their nondescript uniforms were coming in to poke and prod me. They might have been someone's mother, but they weren't mine. And they didn't have my mother's gentleness. Rushing into the room at all hours of the day or night, they brusquely rearranged my blankets, stuffed thermometers in my mouth or jabbed me with needles. On my first visit, they gave me more than twenty-five shots in four days!

I wanted my mother. I'd play the moments of her visits over and over in my mind to soothe myself a bit. I'd remember how she stroked my hair and smiled at me or how she promised to be back the next day. I could see how difficult it was for her to have to go home and leave me in the hospital.

Even though I knew she had to go, the first time she and my father left me there, it was as if something had gone terribly wrong. I had never been separated from my parents for even one night. As soon as I saw my mom pick up her purse, getting ready to leave, I felt a wave of sadness and loneliness come over me. I didn't realize it then, but that sense of melancholy would be with me, one way or another, for many years to come. It was such a horrible experience to be separated from my parents — but especially my mom — that I vowed never to have that experience of desolation again.

Yet, over the next year alone, I'd be back to Children's Hospital in Detroit for surgery several times. My parents had noticed a little red bump under the skin beneath my left eye. After running some tests, the eye doctor diagnosed it as a hemangioma tumor.

Apparently, hemangiomas are very common. Ten percent of all babies have them. Most often, they show up as strawberry birth marks. Some people have them removed and some don't. They're usually benign and not life-threatening unless they appear close to a vital organ. Hemangiomas in the back of the eye can cause blindness. In the lungs, they can attack a child's airways.

My doctor wasn't taking any chances. He recommended we remove it right away. My parents agreed. It was supposed to be a simple, one-time surgery, but it turned out to be more complicated than that.

Two months after the first surgery, the hemangioma grew back. I couldn't believe it. I was still trying to get over my first experience at the hospital when I had to go back to have the tumor removed again! And then it happened again. And again. All in all, I was in surgery four different times to remove the same tumor. It was like a nightmare.

Luckily, when the tumor grew back the third time, my parents took me to another surgeon. He finally removed that little red bump from my face once and for all. But the experience left a lasting impression.

I think there are moments in life that set each of us apart from one another. They are like brightly colored threads in the tapestry of our lives. They may not define us entirely, but they are so interwoven with our sense of ourselves that they become an intricate part of our story.

The first defining moment I remember has to do with kindness.

A surprising feature of my first visit to the hospital was the rule about wheelchairs. The nurse at the front desk told my parents that it was hospital policy for every patient to be taken to their room in a wheelchair. Now that you're our responsibility, we want to make sure that you don't trip and fall (and sue us) is the general idea.

I didn't understand the legal implications as a four-year-old child, but I knew a good ride when I saw one. I hopped into the wheelchair happily and was promptly rolled to the elevator and taken to the highest floor, with my parents tagging along behind. It was like being queen for a day.

When we reached my room, I was in for another surprise. The room was full of cribs! Surely there was some mistake. Didn't this nurse realize what a big girl I was? I hadn't slept in a crib in ages. That was baby stuff. I was way beyond that now.

"It's just to make sure you don't fall out of bed, after surgery," the nurse explained. "We don't want you to get hurt."

To make me feel more at home, she introduced me to all of the girls in the room with me. Most were about my age. A few were even younger. I noticed one of the younger ones with curly blond hair. She sat on her mom's lap, sucking her thumb. I smiled at her and she tried to smile back, but she looked worried. None of us were glad to be there. It was hard enough for me, at my advanced age, but this little girl was only three.

My parents were always so proud of me for being brave during these hospital ordeals. "You're such a big girl," they'd say. "You never cry!"

What they didn't know was that I kept my pain inside, until I was alone in my crib at night. And then I'd cry silently, so the nurses wouldn't hear. I couldn't afford for them to tell my mother. If my mother knew I was crying my heart out every night, missing her so much it hurt, her heart would break.

So I tried to seem brave, but I was faking it — or so I thought.

Now, as an adult, I realize that a good part of bravery is faking it. Being brave means that something scares you, but you do it anyway. At the time, I felt like a four-year-old fake when my parents said I was being brave. What I didn't know was that I wasn't faking it at all. I was brave.

And on that first night, I learned something else. While I was lying there crying, I heard the sound of sniffling from another crib. It was that little blond-haired girl. Because she was younger than I was, I felt like I should do something. I went over and reached my hand between the bars of her crib, gently rubbing her back. My mother always did that to me and I knew it felt good.

"It's all right," I whispered. "Don't cry!" Softly, I started to sing her a song. Before long, she stopped crying and fell asleep.

I did it again, every night I was there. As long I was standing by her crib, singing softly, she fell fast asleep. And it taught me something important: That little bit of kindness helped me too. Giving away comfort, even when you don't have enough, is one of the best ways to comfort yourself.

The second defining moment in the hospital that stands out to me is simpler, but more brightly imprinted on my mind.

It is the day I left the hospital for good.

My parents told me they'd come to pick me up at 11:00 A.M. The nurses didn't need to let me know when that was. At four years old, I already knew how to tell time.

When I woke up that morning, I got dressed, as soon as they'd let me, then I went to the doorway and stood there, like a puppy, waiting happily for my parents. I knew that any second my parents would come around that corner to take me home.

* * *

Once I was safe in the embrace of my parents, the memory of those lonely nights in the hospital receded into the shadows of my mind. Every now and then, when I was alone or awoke from a bad dream, the feeling of lying alone in that hospital room might come back to haunt me. But the rest of my life was so happy, it was easy to believe that nothing like that could ever happen to me again. It seemed like the worst was over.

We were living in Farmington, Michigan, a bedroom community about twenty miles outside of Detroit. With charming Victorian buildings downtown, good schools and lots of parks for kids to play in, it was the perfect place to raise a family. We were living the American dream. My father worked in the family business, an insurance company owned by my grandfather. My mother had her hands full at home, looking after two boys and two girls. Our smiling family photos could've been on a poster for the traditional middle-class family in the sixties. It was one of the happiest times of my life.

When I was ten, I even had a dog follow me home, just like Lassie. So I actually got to say that classic childhood line: "Please, Mom, can I keep her?" Except I had to beg both my parents to let me keep her. I promised that all they'd have to do was buy the dog food and I'd do everything else. I'd make sure she was cleaned and brushed. I'd take her for walks. She'd be my responsibility. They wouldn't have to do a thing. And then, for good measure, I turned on that wide-eyed, pleading look that no loving parent can resist. They didn't stand a chance.

So they reluctantly agreed. Naturally, they warned me that if I didn't take care of her, they'd have to give her away. But I kept my word and took exceptionally good care of my new friend. I called her Shadow and that's what she was. The whole time we were together, we were nearly inseparable. We used to chase each other around the yard or run down the block together,

19

for the sheer joy of running. Sometimes on a Saturday afternoon I'd take her to the park to play fetch, or I'd put her on a leash and take her through the neighborhood, showing her off. Then at night she'd sit by my bed and watch me get situated. When everything was just right, I'd throw back my covers and whisper, "Come on, Shadow!" Getting her cue, she'd jump up on my bed, lie down with her back against my stomach and fall asleep. I'd then throw the covers over the both of us and go to sleep. My mom always said, "Don't let Shadow under the covers!" But I know my mom knew what I was doing and never said a thing.

Shadow was my constant companion. I knew that, no matter what happened to me in my life, I'd never feel lonely as long as I had Shadow.

Everything seemed right with the world in those days. I was well-liked by all my teachers. I had lots of friends. In fact, I was just about the most popular girl in class. I had almost every little girl over to my house to spend the night at least once. And my best friends, Laurie and Cheryl Andrews, were sisters who lived on my street. What could be better?

I can't count the number of happy afternoons I spent with them, talking about school and other kids — especially boys. The popular boys were always interested in me. I even "went steady" with a few of them. Of course, at eleven or twelve, "going steady" meant a boy might hold your hand or if he got up his nerve give you a quick, embarrassed kiss on the cheek before blushing or running away. Whatever happened, Laurie, Cheryl and I would laugh and giggle and tell each other all about it.

I'll never forget the day when the three of us were sitting on the sisters' bedroom floor, in the middle of sixth grade, and suddenly Cheryl said, "You know what? Next year we're all going to go to the same junior high school together. And then we'll go to the same high school after that…"

"Then we'll all pick the same college to go to…" Laurie chimed in.

"And then we'll all get married, have kids and live on the same street," I said, smiling. "We'll be friends for life!"

We were so happy that the best thing we could imagine was to keep things exactly like they were, as much as possible. In the short span of our lives, things had gone so well that there was no reason for us to think that life would ever change. But it did. Almost right away.

* * *

Not long after the sisters and I had planned our perfectly contented lives, my parents dropped a bomb: We were moving to California.

I was devastated. Leave all my friends? I couldn't imagine leaving the neighborhood, much less moving all the way across the country. A few days before, I'd been planning on growing old in Farmington. I could see us trimming Christmas trees at each other's houses with dozens of little grandchildren running around. Didn't they get it? I was going to be happy in Farmington for the rest of my life. Why on earth would I want to move to California? Who would do such a thing?

I pleaded with my parents to let us stay in Michigan. Things wouldn't be the same in California, I knew it. It would be a terrible decision to move. I gave them all the reasons an impassioned twelve-year-old could come up with.

Little did I know it, but I was too late. My dad had already taken a job in Ojai, about forty-five miles from Santa Barbara, teaching at a private high school. He wanted to get out of the insurance business and said it would be good for all of us to start a new life.

My parents talked about how sunny and beautiful it was in California. They told us how much we'd like our new schools and said we wouldn't even have to wear our big coats and boots in the winter because it was so warm there all year round. But none of that mattered. It saddened me immensely to be yanked away from my friends and the life I loved. I wanted things to stay just as they were.

I seemed to be the only one in the family who felt that way.

My younger sister and brother weren't old enough to care. David had only been born the year before and was still in diapers. He was in no position to argue. Julie was six years old and as long as she was with the family she'd be happy anywhere. And Craig, my older brother, was excited about going to California. All the beach movies in the sixties were set in California and then there were cool TV shows like *Sunset Strip*, where good-looking guys would ride along the beach in their convertibles, surrounded by beautiful girls in bikinis. For a young teenage boy, it must've sounded like he was being asked to move to heaven.

Still, it sounded like the end of the world to me. After my arguments gave out, I put my arms around Shadow for solace and buried my face in her furry neck. They might be able to force me to move, but I made up my mind to resist it every step of the way.

And then the real bomb hit.

"Oh," my mother said. "There's one more thing… We're not going to be buying a house in California at first. We're going to be renting. We've already put down a deposit for the first year, so we can't back out now, but …" Kind hearted as she was, she couldn't bear to say it. So she glanced at my father for support.

"There are no pets allowed," he said.

I could hardly believe it. First they asked me to give up everything I knew — my life and all my friends. Now I was going to have to leave my dog behind too? It was too much to bear. The thought of losing Shadow was even worse than moving to California. If I had been able to take the dog, it would have been so much easier for me to make the transition. Without her, it would be horrible. I would have nothing to comfort me.

After that I felt numb. Even though my life had been happy, it had still had its ups and downs. I had always been a sensitive child, responding to things with emotion that didn't seem to bother other kids. Already there were signs of tension between my parents. No one had said anything, but they didn't have to. Children always sense the emotional strain. And, in my case, I turned to my dog for consolation. For all my popularity at school and my closeness to the Andrews girls, I found my deepest emotional comfort in my Shadow.

Leaving my dog behind was the most distressing thing I'd ever been through. As a child, it consumed me. From the day I was told I couldn't take her with me, until long after we had moved to California, the loss hung like a grim, black cloud over my head. It saddened me as nothing ever had.

Sitting on the front steps with my arm around her neck, in the days before we left, I thought about running away with Shadow. But where do young girls run to when they run away? We could go hide in the park for a couple of hours or so, but it would get cold after dark and we wouldn't have anything to eat. It's not like there were little houses set up on the outskirts of town for runaway girls and their dogs.

"I would do it!" I swore to Shadow, squeezing her tight. "Don't think I wouldn't!" But the truth was, I didn't know where we could go. So I guessed that idea was out.

Unbelievable as it seemed, my perfect life was coming to an end. And there was nothing I could do to stop it. None of it was under my control. I was being dragged away from the things I cared about most. Very soon I was going to be alone, without my home, my friends or my dog for comfort. And I desperately needed comfort. So I started to binge.

2

Weighing In

How does it feel to be fat? Is it something you think about every day or only some of the time? What difference does it make in your life?

Looking back on it now, I can tell you that it was a miserable experience. I thought about it all the time. When I walked into a room and people innocently glanced up at me, I'd tell myself, "They're thinking how fat I am." When someone rejects you or doesn't like you, you blame yourself for being fat. Even if you're only a little chubby, the extra weight you carry can change your life.

It's difficult at any age, but being overweight as a kid is especially hard. Most kids are self-conscious anyway. They're always trying to figure out where they fit in. They're focused on being accepted, not on being themselves. They want to find other kids like them to be a part of the group. If you're fat, you aren't like the other kids … not the cool ones anyway. You're different. And you're made to feel bad about it. The fatter you are, the harder it is to feel accepted and loved.

We all have embarrassing memories from our childhoods. But when you're overweight, some of your most humiliating memories are about being fat.

* * *

Two of my earliest embarrassments happened even before we left Michigan. I remember playing in my bedroom in

Farmington one day when I heard my grandmother's voice in the kitchen. She was in the kitchen with my mom. I was very fond of Grandma, so I stopped what I was doing and went down the hall toward the kitchen to see her.

When I came out of my room, I thought I heard her mention my name. She was talking softly, so as not to be heard. As I moved down the hall, I heard my mom say my name too. Now I was really interested in what they were saying! I started to tiptoe as I approached the door, leaning forward so I could hear...

"Are you sure?" Grandma whispered, urgently.

My mom sounded kind of defensive. "Yes, Mother, I'm sure," she said. "I should know..." I could hear from Mom's voice that she didn't want to be having this conversation with her mother.

What were they talking about? As quietly as I could, I slowly pulled the swinging door to the kitchen open — just a crack — so I could hear what they were saying.

"Maybe it's something she gets at school, "my grandma said. "Do you think that's it?"

"I don't know," my mom muttered. "I see what she eats here... and I don't think it's too much."

I started to have a queasy feeling. They were talking about me. But they were talking about the one thing I didn't want to hear!

Then Grandma said it: "She's gained quite a bit of weight since I saw her last time. It isn't healthy." You could hear the tsk-tsk-tsk! of condemnation in her voice. "She must be getting food from other places besides home."

Now she was making me out to be some sort of thief, sneaking around, snatching up food anywhere I could get it. In a year or two, that's exactly what I would be doing, but I wasn't doing it then. The idea hadn't even occurred to me yet.

At the time, I was just embarrassed — for me and my mother — and sorry I'd eavesdropped. As I gently closed the door, trying not to make a sound, I heard my mom say, "Well, if that's what she's doing, then there's nothing I can do about it." She sounded miserable. I felt exactly the same way.

As I snuck quietly back to my bedroom, the thought hit me: My own grandma sees me as an overweight kid. I'd always thought I was one of her favorites. Now I realized that she was probably embarrassed by me — her only fat grandchild. It was a rude awakening.

When Grandma called out to me before she left that day, I ignored her and pretended that I didn't hear. I wasn't as excited about seeing her after that because I wanted her to just leave me alone. In my heart, I was always glad to see her, but I couldn't forget what she'd said.

Whether or not my grandma ever felt anything like what I assumed she felt, it was one of the first times that my weight had made me feel trapped and cut off from love.

* * *

After that, the embarrassing moment that stands out most in my mind happened in sixth grade gym class and it was a lot more complex.

Since the weather in Michigan isn't good for much of the year, we usually had our daily P.E. class in the gymnasium at my elementary school. I loved P.E. and I was very good at sports. Volleyball was my favorite. I once won a ribbon for being on the best team in class. Sports always gave me the feeling of being vigorous and alive.

The only thing I dreaded about P.E. was the one day a year when we all had to be weighed and measured. It was mandatory. Some state regulation. Thank God it was only once a year.

Throughout grade school, I was never as small and thin as the other little girls. I was always around five to ten pounds heavier than the others, but, as my mom pointed out, I was one of the tallest girls in the class, too. She liked to say I wasn't really chubby. I was "solid."

The truth is, I knew I was a few pounds overweight and it bothered me, but I had no idea what to do about it. My best solution was to hang out with a girl who really was chubby. Even as a young girl, I figured that hanging out with someone fatter than myself could only help me look good.

My other strategy was temporary. When it came time for us to be weighed and measured, Mr. Adams, our P.E. teacher, would sometimes let us know the day before. If I knew we were going to be weighed, I'd skip lunch that day and drink a small milk, hoping to be a little bit lighter.

For a couple of years I had a bit of a crush on Mr. Adams. He reminded me of my dad because he was a tall man, about 6'4", and had a deep, powerful voice. Like a typical coach, he always wore gym clothes and had a whistle around his neck. He was pretty nice to us in general, unless one of the boys acted out and that's when he got tough.

Because I liked him and wanted to impress him, the way this whole weighing incident turned out was especially painful. It didn't help that my arch nemesis, Jeannine, was involved.

Every year, Mr. Adams would ask for a volunteer to record the height and weight of each student. Most of the time he chose Jeannine. She was clearly the teacher's pet.

Many of the girls in my class didn't like her. Jeannine was too competitive. She wanted so badly to be the best and most popular student in class. But that year, it had gotten personal, after I'd won the spelling bee. Jeannine had been so disappointed to lose that she'd actually started crying on the way back to her desk. And I'd felt sorry for her. But not for long.

A few weeks later Jeannine had her revenge. Mr. Adams announced that it was time for us to be weighed and measured. And, naturally, Jeannine was chosen as the volunteer to take our weight and measurements. She took everyone's weight and measurements carefully. She didn't give anything away. Except, when I stepped on the scale, I saw her smile. More of a smirk, really, and it didn't bode well.

Later that day, I saw Jeannine talking to a few of the girls in class after everyone had been weighed and felt the same uneasy feeling that I'd felt when I heard my grandma in the kitchen. People were whispering about my weight again.

I forced myself to walk over to the group, but they all stopped talking when they saw me. Then suddenly, my own friend, Sarah, taunted me, in a cruel, sing-songy voice, "I know what you weigh!" And all three of them giggled, ridiculing me. I couldn't help it. I burst into tears. And I went to find Mr. Adams, because I knew this wasn't right.

When he saw me crying, Mr. Adams was concerned at first. He got up from his chair and came over to put his hand on my shoulder, like my dad, and asked me what was wrong.

"Jeannine told the other girls what I weigh and now they're all making fun of me!" I sobbed, hanging my head.

I could feel his hand go cold on my shoulder. I'd expected Jeannine to get in trouble, but when I looked up, I could see this wasn't going to happen. Mr. Adams didn't believe me. "Jeannine wouldn't do that," was all he said.

There was no point discussing it. The coach had called the game.

When someone embarrasses you about being fat, one of the worst things of all is the sense of futility. There's no point discussing it. When my grandma and Jeannine were whispering that I was fat, I felt humiliated. But I secretly thought they were right. So what could I say, "I'm really not fat"? It's futile. You're trapped.

How does it feel to be fat?

It feels bad. Every day.

* * *

I guess that explains why I started stealing.

Not everyone would start stealing in response to the embarrassments and humiliations of their life. And maybe that's not why I did it either. But it's as good an explanation as any.

I started out stealing dessert, then worked my way up to valuable merchandise.

Dessert at our house was usually two cookies — not one cookie, not three cookies — but two cookies. My dad thought two cookies was exactly the right amount and wouldn't let me have any more.

But I wanted more. So I learned to be a thief.

After everyone had gone to bed, I'd sneak back into the kitchen, quietly open the cupboard and carefully slide the pack of cookies out. It took a special skill not to make a sound with the rumpled paper with my heart pounding like it was.

Once I had the bag open, I'd grab five or six cookies and cram them into my pocket, then casually stroll to the bathroom, lock the door and eat the cookies as fast as I could. What a rush! It had it all — the excitement of sneaking into the kitchen at night, the thrill of stealing something I wasn't supposed to have, the fear of getting caught — not to mention the sudden infusion of sugar in my blood. It didn't take me long to realize that food tasted better when I stole it.

I liked it so much that when we moved to California I started doing it in the kitchen of my new best friend.

* * *

When I saw the house my parents had rented in Santa Barbara, I had to admit it was very cool. It was on a hill at the end of a cul-de-sac with a steep, private driveway. We had a view of the Pacific Ocean from our living room and a view of the Santa Ynez Mountains out the back. But I wasn't letting my parents off the hook that easily. They'd taken my friends and my dog away from me. I was pretty sure I'd be lonely for the rest of my life and it was their fault.

While they were unpacking, I took my bike out to the driveway and rode around, with as much attitude as I could muster. My sulky look was like an accusation: "I will never be happy here!"

And then something unexpected happened. Over at the end of our property, I saw a girl my age throwing her leg over the fence to come into our yard. I stopped my bike and stared at her.

"Hi!" she said. "My name's Kristy Wagner."

As it turned out, we were in the same grade and she lived one street over from us. Kristy truly made living in California easier for me. She was my first new friend and the only friend I really had for several years.

With Kristy, I didn't feel so lonely anymore, although I thought about my friends back home every day. Laurie and Cheryl and I had promised to write to each other and never stop. My other friends were determined to write too. We all kept it up for about a year, but inevitably we lost contact.

In many ways, it was a sad time for me. California itself was a much happier, more beautiful place than I could've imagined as a child in Michigan, but my feeling of foreboding about the move was turning out to be right. I was much less happy here than I had been in Farmington. The loss of my close companion, Shadow, was a constant pocket of sorrow in my heart. And, as much as I liked Kristy, I missed the joy of going to a school every day where I had lots and lots of friends.

At this new school, I felt shy and it was harder for me to make as many new friends. I was quiet and uncertain. I liked eating lunch with Kristy at school, if I could find her, but when I couldn't I'd eat alone on the lawn.

I felt overly self-conscious sitting alone all by myself. My only solution was to try to build a wall around myself, then I wouldn't have to worry about what the other kids were saying or thinking about me. If they did make a mean remark, I didn't have the nerve to say anything back.

Being shy was actually a way to get respect from people, in some ways. Parents and teachers tend to like shy, bright, young girls. And I was almost a straight "A" student, so that helped.

* * *

The downside of my being shy was that I didn't have the gumption to stand up for myself when I needed to, like when our neighbor next door in Michigan began to molest me. I knew I didn't like it, but I was too shy to open my mouth and tell that evil man to stop doing those horrible things to me. So I endured his molesting for two whole years.

Mom and Dad didn't know our neighbor Mr. Thomas well, yet he was still considered a friend of the family. He had a wife and two sons. His wife was in sales and would often be away on business. His sons were away at school.

They had a large garden in their backyard. Mr. Thomas was retired and spent a lot of his time gardening. From the large picture window in our house, I watched Mr. Thomas gardening and mowing the lawn, and if he saw me looking at him, he'd wave to me.

One day while my mother was out on errands, Mr. Thomas called to me and asked, "Would you like to come over to my house and pick some vegetables for your family?"

I said, "Okay," and told the babysitter I'd be up the street with Mr. Thomas. Back in the sixties there were no worries about the neighbors. The neighborhoods felt safe. Mr. Thomas showed me around his garden and told me what each vegetable was and how to know when they were ready for picking. As he talked about his garden, often he would hug me or kiss my cheek. I didn't like it. It was different when my dad did it. Being shy, though, I couldn't tell him to stop. As I left with my pickings, Mr. Thomas said, "Come back again soon, dear." I smiled bashfully and ran home, glad to be away from him.

A few days later, just after mom left to do errands, the phone rang and I answered. It was Mr. Thomas again. "I was wondering if you'd like to come over to pick vegetables again."

"My mom isn't here right now so I can't."

Mr. Thomas replied, "Just ask your babysitter. Fresh vegetables for your family dinner tonight. Your mom will love it!"

Too timid to argue, I asked the babysitter and she said yes. She even gave me a bag to put the vegetables in. As I crossed our front yard and got close to his front door, I saw Mr. Thomas standing in his living room as he watched my every step. It gave me the creeps. He motioned for me to go around to the side of the house where the garage was, so I walked over to the side of the house. He opened the garage door to let me in, and then closed it behind me.

"I thought you might be interested in seeing a gift I've bought for Mrs. Thomas, he said. "It's a secret and only you and I will know what it is."

I didn't like the garage door being down. I was waiting to see what Mrs. Thomas's gift was, but Mr. Thomas started talking about something else and I never did get to see it. He talked about boring things, but I listened attentively and tried to show interest. I had been taught to be polite to adults and, when they talked, to respect and listen to them.

Four steps led from the garage into the house, and Mr. Thomas sat on the top step, gently pulling me over to him so that I was standing between his legs and we were eye-to-eye. As he talked, he kept gently rubbing my arms and back. Every time he said something he thought was funny and I'd laugh, he'd hold my head in his hands and kiss my cheeks several times.

A few days later, Mr. Thomas again called to invite me over to pick vegetables, telling me to just meet him in his garage. He was sitting on the steps waiting for me, a big smile on his face. When he pulled down the garage door, I said, "I don't like the garage door down."

"It's cold in here. I don't want you to be cold," he said. He seemed to make all the decisions. Every time I showed up at his house, he would get bolder with me. One day while he and I were in the garage — always with the garage door down — he slowly put his hands down my pants and started to rub my private parts and bottom. He did this for several minutes, all the while chitchatting about trivial things to distract me from what he was actually doing to me.

This molesting went on for about two years and, after a while, he would even call when my mom was home, having figured out I hadn't told my parents what was going on in his garage.

It seems odd to me now, as an adult, why I never discussed this with my mom since we were so close, but it never came up. I doubted my feelings. I always endured my visits with Mr. Thomas, but I thought this was a nice man who knew my parents. I simply could not have conceived that Mr. Thomas or any adult could be doing something wrong.

I did tell my brother, Craig, soon after the last incident happened. Craig didn't believe me at the time. I slowly forgot about it.

Apparently, Craig told my mom years later, because I was too embarrassed to tell her myself. When she tried to bring the subject up years later with me, she apologized for not realizing anything so horrible was happening to me. Then she told Dad. His reaction was, "I wish you would have told me about Mr. Thomas when this was going on because I would have…." And he pounded his fist into the palm of his other hand. And my dad isn't a violent man.

The molesting had taken place during a difficult period. On top of our moving to California, to make matters worse, our family was breaking up. Apparently, my parents hadn't told us everything about the move. We did live in a great house in Santa Barbara, but my dad lived in Ojai, in an apartment near the school where he was teaching. We hardly ever saw him.

This move wasn't just about a new job or a change of scenery. My parents were separated.

* * *

I was so embarrassed that we didn't have a "normal" family, that I kept it a secret, even from my only friend. Kristy's parents were happily married. So I acted like mine were too, except my father had to stay out of town to work. Ojai was only a forty-five minute commute from Santa Barbara, but Kristy seemed to buy it.

With my father gone, there was a thin, gray fog of depression over my house for ages. It was much happier at Kristy's house. I practically lived over there. Sometimes I'd even pretend that I was one of Kristy's sisters.

Besides, Mrs. Wagner let us eat whatever we wanted. She always told me to help myself to any of their food while I was over. How cool was that!

I took advantage of it too. My cookie-stealing days were back. Once everyone in the house was asleep, I'd wake up in the middle of the night and sneak down into the kitchen. Mrs. Wagner bought different cookies than my mom did and, boy, were they good! Usually, she had several different kinds. I'd quietly uncurl the bags and swipe a few cookies of each kind. Then I'd devour them quickly and hurry back to bed.

Since Mrs. Wagner had said I could have them, it didn't have quite the same rush as disobeying my dad, but no one knew I'd taken them. So it still felt like I was getting away with something.

After carefully wiping the cookie crumbs from my face, I'd slip back into bed next to Kristy and pull the covers up to my chin, lying very still, listening for any noise. If someone got up right away, it might mean they'd heard me rummaging around the kitchen. So I'd wait, with my heart pounding... but there was never a sound.

The greatest high would come when I knew — actually knew for sure — that I'd gotten away with it. After that I could go to sleep with a satisfied smile on my face.

Stealing was my one private pleasure. And it was a total rush. I had to go further. If it was this much fun to steal cookies from the kitchen, what would it be like to steal something from a store?

3

My Biggest Year

STEALING FROM DEPARTMENT STORES TURNED OUT TO BE even more of a thrill than I'd expected.

When I was sneaking into the kitchen late at night to steal food, I wasn't in any real danger. Not only did I have the benefit of darkness, but I was surrounded by people I knew. If Kristy's mom had woken up and caught me shoving cookies into my mouth, it would've been embarrassing, but she wouldn't have called the police.

When I stole clothes from a department store, I was committing a crime among total strangers in broad daylight. They would've been only too happy to turn me into the police if they'd had any idea what I was doing. It was a tremendous thrill.

Stealing things got rid of my depression almost instantly. And it wasn't even fattening.

Sometimes I'd steal because I was just mad at everything and stealing helped alleviate the pressure. Other times I'd steal for the high. It was like taking a drug. As soon as it wore off, I'd go back out to the stores to steal something again.

Like most shoplifters I could easily afford most of the things I took. I had a babysitting job and made about twenty-five dollars a week. So I had more than enough money to buy what I wanted. In fact, sometimes I didn't even want it.

I'd go into a dressing room to try things on, without finding anything I liked, but I would steal something anyway — just because I could. I loved the feeling that I was outsmarting the stores. Every time I passed one of those stuffy, condescending store clerks in the ladies' clothes department, with a blouse or skirt tucked secretly away under my clothes, I couldn't help but repress a little smile.

It was the same thing I'd felt the first time I stole cookies from the cupboard when everybody else was asleep: I was getting away with something. But stealing from the stores was so much better.

Over the years, I stole a lot of merchandise. For awhile, when I was thirteen, I focused on gum. Don't ask me why, but at some point I'd decided to make a gum wrapper chain thirty feet long. It was going to take a hundreds of packs of gum to do that. So I had to get busy. There was a lot of work ahead. In a single afternoon, I would go to four or five different stores, slipping a few packets of gum from each one into my pocket, to build up my collection. Before long, I'd stolen so much gum I had to give it away.

Once my gum chain was complete, I started getting bolder. By the time I was fourteen, I was stealing clothes from stores on a regular basis. Before long, I realized I was getting pretty good at this and would probably never get caught.

At the end of the day, I'd go home and add everything up. I'd write the total in my journal at the bottom of the page. I never wrote anything about stealing. There was just this mysterious number on page after page — in case anyone, like my mother, got a hold of it. On December 31 of that year, my total was 450 dollars. I couldn't help but feel proud.

My journals were filled with entries about dieting and losing weight, but curiously enough I never wrote down what I ate. Most of the pages were filled with comments about how I was going to go on a diet — "tomorrow FOR SURE" — or how tired I was of being overweight. I would make endless lists of reasons why I HAD TO lose weight as if all I needed to do was to persuade myself. Those pages were usually followed by curt, dismissive notes that just said: "Blew it" or "Start tomorrow" or "Good until noon, then blew it again."

Looking back on it now, it's easy for me to see that I was just trying to find comfort or reprieve wherever I could. By thirteen years old, I felt like giving up on life. We had left my dog and a life I loved behind to come to a place where I was miserably unhappy. My parents weren't getting along, so there was tension in the house. And to make things worse, I was being picked on at school for being fat. Even Kristy's brother made "oinking" noises when I walked by.

In Michigan, I'd been popular and happy at school. For all I knew, my parents had been happy too. The world had seemed just right to me there. Now, nothing was going my way. It made me angry. And I wanted somebody to pay. What I didn't see for the longest time was that I was the one who was paying the price.

* * *

And then one day, things got even worse. I was lying on my bed, listening to my Cher albums when my mom came in, holding a cup of tea for comfort.

"Your dad and I are getting a divorce, Linda," she said, as gently as she could. "We've filed the paperwork. It's going to be final soon."

I didn't see this coming. Well maybe I did, but I didn't want to admit it. I never thought of asking Mom or Dad about their marriage and they never shared any details about their marriage with us at the time. I didn't say a word and hoped for the best. But the best wasn't going to happen. They were getting a divorce.

Something inside of me froze. I didn't want to hear this. If I could just keep staring at the ceiling and focus on the music, maybe I could make the whole thing go away. I lay there, not moving a muscle, doing my best to blot my mother out. How could she and my dad do this to me? They'd already taken me away from my home and everything I loved. Now this? I felt betrayed.

I hadn't said a word, but she could see how badly I was taking it. There was nothing she could say to make things better, but my mom did her best. "I was thinking that we could all go to the pound to pick out a puppy," she said, hopefully. "What do you think?"

My eyes welled up with tears, but I wouldn't let them fall in front of my mom. She felt like the enemy to me then.

Gradually, it dawned on her that I wasn't going to speak and she quietly left the room. I jumped up quickly and locked the door, then did what countless kids in my generation did in a moment like that. I went to the record player and put on the heartbreaking song that Sonny wrote when he was getting a divorce from Cher: "You Better Sit Down Kids." I played the song over and over again that day, crying into my pillow so no one would hear.

* * *

After that, I stopped talking to my mom for about a year. I don't mean I gave her attitude or answered her in grunts and monosyllables like some teenagers do half the time anyway. I completely stopped talking.

She had ruined my life and I wanted to punish her. When I thought of the cruelest thing I could do, that was it. She'd ask me questions and I wouldn't answer her. We never had conversations.

Now and then, as I walked out the door, at most, I'd mutter, in a grumpy voice, "I'm going out." If she wanted to know when I'd be back or if I'd pick up some milk for the family while I was out, she was out of luck. I never answered. I'd just shut the door and leave.

My father had given my brother and me the impression that the divorce was my mom's fault, so I blamed her. I really believed as only an angry adolescent can that if I didn't talk to her, Mom might "wise up," see the damage she was causing and get back together with my dad.

Of course, years later, I found out that the real story was somewhat different than I'd been told. Before we'd even left Michigan, my dad had told my mom he wanted a different life and he was moving to California. In an effort to keep the family together, my mom said we would move to California too. But I didn't know that at the time. And, as the months rolled by, my sullenness began to get to my mom.

I can only imagine the kind of pain and fear she was going through at the time. Her life had been uprooted too. She had wanted to keep her marriage together and had moved all the way across the country to do it, but it had failed anyway. With the disappointment of loss and the pressure of starting a new life as a single parent, it must have been intense. The last thing she needed was more punishment from me for something she'd tried to prevent.

One morning, she had had all she could take. I was sitting at the breakfast table having breakfast when she came into the room.

There was tension in her voice when she spoke. "Linda, I can't find the paper. Did you take it from the front lawn?"

I didn't answer her. I just kept eating my cereal.

To my surprise, she raised her voice, then came toward me and hit me on the head. "I asked you a question and I expect you to answer. Did you get the paper?!"

"No!" I yelled, then got up from the table and ran to my bedroom. I slammed the door and cried. It was one of the few times Mom ever scared me, but I truly deserved it.

* * *

I was so embarrassed about the divorce that I didn't tell Kristy. I continued to keep up the ruse that my parents were just living apart for awhile because my father had to work far away. I kept the secret for years after the divorce was final, suffering the humiliation of my broken family in secret.

40

The irony is that, when I finally did tell Kristy, she didn't think it was a shameful secret at all. She said something like, "Oh, that's too bad. I like your parents. They're cool," and then she changed the subject. I could have saved myself a lot of misery by confiding in Kristy early on, especially since, for a few years, Kristy was my only friend.

I was shy and unpopular until I was about fifteen. Then one day, it occurred to me that I was missing out on much of life by being shy. I literally made a decision to stop being shy and introverted. "From now on, I'm going to be open and talkative," I told myself. "I'll be an extrovert."

I'd always had a good sense of humor. I'd been far too shy to say the funny things that were running through my head. Now, I decided to start muttering those little smart aleck remarks aloud. And people laughed. They liked me and thought I was funny.

In no time at all, I went from being terribly shy, to being the opposite — loud, gregarious, joking around a lot. Before long, I was considered the class clown.

* * *

With my new popularity, I was hanging out with a lot of new friends. And in high school, that means it's only a matter of time before someone introduces you to cigarettes.

One night I went to visit my friend Elizabeth at a restaurant where she worked. When we went outside on her break, she pulled out a pack of cigarettes and offered me one. I felt very, very cool as Elizabeth lit my cigarette. From watching movies, I knew how to hold it between my fingers and take a slow, sophisticated puff.

I didn't know I'd gag and start coughing!

Why would anybody smoke? I thought, looking at the cigarette in horror.

Elizabeth laughed. "You know, you'll lose weight if you

start smoking. When you get hungry, you can smoke instead of eating."

I bought a pack that night and never quit smoking for twenty-eight years.

The next morning, when I got up, I took my cup of coffee outside to drink it with a cigarette. In my new life as a popular outgoing girl, I'd recently started drinking coffee too. And everyone talked about the wonderful combination of coffee and cigarettes. I could hardly wait to try it. But it made me nauseous.

"Just keep at it," Elizabeth told me. "You'll get used to it."

Strange as it seems now, I was determined to keep smoking no matter what, even though it was making me sick and the smoke was giving me coughing fits. I hoped it would help me lose weight, but more importantly it was part of my new, improved life — something I could call my own.

* * *

From my point of view, my life was starting to look up. When I bought my first car at sixteen, things got even better. Sometimes it seemed like everything I did was constrained by other people — what they liked and how they thought things should be done. With a car, I could go where I wanted and do the things I liked to do. My depression was gone. I was much happier at school. And I started spending more time with Denise, one of my new friends. I liked Denise because I could say anything I wanted to her. She was a great listener and always gave me her undivided attention. We used to go out for dinner every Friday night and sit and talk for hours.

For awhile, I felt especially comfortable with Denise because she loved to eat like I did. But then she went on a crash diet. In three months, she lost fifty pounds. She still went out to dinner with me, but it wasn't as comfortable as before.

Now Denise was sitting there, several sizes smaller, looking thin and drinking black coffee, while I was chugging down my patty melts with French fries and strawberry shakes. I felt envious of her success in losing weight, but I knew I was a lot more popular than she was and much more outgoing, so I didn't feel too bad and we managed to stay good friends.

Despite my overall happiness, I was still gaining a lot of weight. At first, it was all I could do to squeeze into size sixteen jeans. When I couldn't wear those anymore, I switched to dresses. I adamantly refused to buy size eighteen jeans, though now and then, I secretly bought my dresses in maternity shops.

As long as I was dieting, it was easier to believe the extra weight was just a temporary thing. On the days I stuck to my diet, I felt stronger and happier than on the days when I overate. But that didn't keep me from cheating.

Eventually that year, I got up to my highest weight, 210 pounds. At sixteen years old, I was seventy-five pounds overweight. I wrote in my journal: "I feel like a fat slob."

4

A Defining Moment

I USED TO FANTASIZE ABOUT BEING ABLE TO CONTROL MY eating. I'd have imaginary conversations with myself, where someone would ask me, "Would you like another chocolate chip cookie?"

And I'd reply, politely, "No, thank you. I'm too full."

It was comforting to imagine I had self-control. But I rather doubted I could ever achieve it in real life. So many people — including my entire family! — could just stop eating when they were full. They could be satisfied with just one cookie. But I was never satisfied. I was like a bottomless pit. And I hated it.

I wanted to be able to honestly say "no, thank you" and mean it some day, but just thinking about turning down cookies was enough to make me dig out the stash of Chips Ahoy I kept hidden underneath my clothes in the top drawer. I'd sit on my bed, eating one after another until I couldn't cram any more cookies into my mouth. My stomach felt like it was going to explode. Stop at one cookie? I wouldn't think of it. I could easily devour twenty cookies at a time. I'd feel this rush of anticipation and then it was as if something took me over and I just started gobbling them down. I couldn't stop myself.

Whenever I went to the shopping center, I'd bring home bags of sweetness — cookies, candy bars, Twinkies, whatever I could find — and keep them hidden, like a private consolation that no one else could take away. I could easily eat several candy bars at a time: Hershey Bars, Baby Ruth, Butterfinger,

Snickers and Nestle's bars — those were my favorite. I thought of food as comfort, but it wasn't like I enjoyed eating it.

Behind my closed bedroom door, I could eat as fast and sloppily as I wanted. I could stuff the food into my mouth without anyone correcting me or making snide remarks. I loved the sugar high that followed, but the truth is, I barely tasted the food as I was shoveling it into my mouth.

Don't get me wrong, the Twinkies, vanilla ice cream and chocolate chip cookies, all tasted great, but it wasn't about taste. And it wasn't about hunger. I was feeding something else in the privacy of my room. But the effects were very public.

In four years, I gained ninety pounds.

By the time I graduated high school, I'd been on one crash diet after another. My favorite was the Dr. Stillman Diet that was so popular at the time. But I tried anything to lose weight: fasting, Slim Wrap and not eating after twelve noon. I'd been on a five-hundred-calorie-a-day diet and the high-protein diet my doctor had used to lose one hundred pounds.

In between candy bars and bags of Chips Ahoy, I'd been battling my weight with diets for years, going on and coming off of them very quickly. I'd stick to a diet for about three days, gorge myself on the fourth day, then get right back on the diet the day after.

Wanting to look good for graduation photos, I somehow managed to keep the gorging to a minimum toward the end of high school. After staying on a low-carb diet for several months, I managed to lose thirty-eight pounds by graduation.

When you lose almost forty pounds, it makes a huge difference. Instead of looking fat at graduation, I looked "big." I weighed 172 and couldn't seem to go any lower. At 5'9" the weight charts said I should weigh between 139 and 153. I'd gone from being clearly obese to being overweight. And that was no small feat.

But I still hated the fact that I could do so well for days, then I'd feel that adrenalin rush again and something would come over me. I'd lose control and binge. At that rate, I couldn't seem to get below 172. Every time I'd start to make progress, I'd lose control and gain the weight back.

By October of 1974, I was feeling frustrated and trapped. I knew that I could never really be thin if I couldn't stay in control of my eating. But I didn't know what else to do.

* * *

In the back of my mind, I kept thinking of something my dad had said months before. I'd made some comment about being overweight and he said he knew the secret to losing weight for good. I was hoping it would be a wonderful new diet, something like: "Eat all the chocolate chip cookies you want and still lose weight!"

But when we finally sat down to talk about it, my dad told me that the secret to losing weight was to turn it over to God. "It's the only way you'll have a true healing of your weight problem," he assured me.

Turning it over to God didn't mean much to me at the time. I had grown up believing in God. And my dad said that, even as a child, I'd been "a very spiritual being," but I'd never felt that close to God.

My dad hadn't seemed especially close to God either, until he'd had an accident several years before, when we were living in Michigan.

It was winter and the streets were slick with ice, as he walked back to work after lunch. Just as he reached his office, he slipped on the ice and fell forward, face down, on the pavement. He hit the ground so hard, it nearly knocked him out. As he lay there, half-conscious, the secretaries in his office came running out to see if he was all right. One of them asked if she could contact a Christian Science practitioner on his behalf. Lying on the pavement, cold, afraid and in pain, my dad agreed.

At the time, he wasn't even sure if he was okay and didn't know what his face looked like. But within moments, he began to feel a gentle peace fill his body. It gradually rose up to his face and he sensed that he was somehow being healed. By the next day, instead of the swelling and bruising he expected after such a horrendous fall, it was difficult to tell that anything had happened.

He was so curious about the experience that, when he learned that the secretary had called a Christian Science practitioner in Chicago, he booked a flight and went to meet her.

"It's a miracle," he told the practitioner. "By the morning after the accident, my face was completely healed. What did you do?"

The woman smiled and said, "In God's kingdom, there are no accidents."

The experience had a tremendous impact on my dad. In the years that followed, he had continued searching to find out what God and Spirit really meant. He hadn't talked a lot about it at the time, but I do remember one day, when he said, "Linda, there really is a God" and it stuck.

I'd never thought of God as the answer to my weight problem, until my dad had mentioned it. Even when he said it, I didn't believe anything would come of asking God for help, but it was starting to become clear that I had absolutely nothing to lose.

* * *

On October 5, 1974, I was sitting in my room on a Saturday night at about seven-thirty. I'd already eaten dinner, so I wasn't very hungry, but I craved something sweet. So I took out the large bag of M&M's I had hidden away in my drawer.

At first, I poured a small handful of M&M's into my mouth and ate them. Then I neatly folded the wrapping paper down and put the candy back in the drawer.

It was a good moment. I was practicing the self-control I'd fantasized about so many times. I told myself I didn't crave anything else. I felt satisfied. If someone had asked, "Would you like a few more M&M's?" I could've said, "No, thanks. I'm full." There was no reason to eat any more that night and I knew it.

I was in such a good mood that I put on a Sonny and Cher album. Dancing and lip syncing to a Cher album was one of my favorite things to do. I used to grow my hair and nails long to look like Cher's. It was so easy to see myself as Cher — a tall, thin, glamorous rock star with that deeply resonant voice.

For awhile, I danced around the room with my hair brush as a microphone, lip syncing along to one of her classics. I'd just about perfected the way she swung her hair around, when she turned to Sonny and sang, as they grinned together:

I got you, babe!
I got you, babe!

And I knew just where to chime in with Cher when they took turns on the lines. It was like I was belting it out next to Sonny myself.

I got you to hold my hand
I got you to understand...

I was just where I wanted to be — completely lost in Cher's world, up on the stage like Cher, looking like Cher, singing like Cher, living Cher's life ... but in some other part of my mind, I was back in my own world and my thoughts kept returning to that open bag of candy in the drawer ...

I got you to kiss goodnight...

I could still taste the chocolate on my lips.

I got you to hold me tight...

I had most of the bag left. And my stomach was starting to feel kind of empty, in a way...

I got you, I won't let go
I got you...

Before I knew it, I had opened the drawer again and taken out that bag of M&M's. God, why did I keep obsessing over this? Why couldn't I just enjoy what I was doing — listening to records — and not have to think about food? Did I really need this? Couldn't I just stop now and put the candy back in the drawer?

I was so determined to finally take control of my life that I did just that.

I did it to prove to myself I actually could take control. It was easy. I just folded back the wrapper, put the candy under my shirts and closed the drawer. There. That's all it took. Was that so hard?

Cher had moved on to her next song. But I was too distracted to sync along. I lay down on my bed, trying to listen, unable to let go of my thoughts about the candy. Had I really conquered my compulsion? Was this the night that I was going to succeed in exerting my willpower and taking control of food?

I truly didn't know at first. Then there it was again — that old familiar feeling of adrenaline, surging throughout my body. I got off the bed, as if in a trance, and headed for the drawer.

A sickening feeling of failure swept over me, but I kept going. I was starting to feel angry too. How could I let myself down like this? How could I give in when I'd been so close to succeeding?

I just don't care, I told myself, fending off my anger. I want this chocolate.

I opened the bag and poured as much candy into my

hand as it could hold. Then I tossed back my head and threw it into my mouth, chewing, frantically. I threw another handful of candy into my mouth, then another. I was on a roll. I wouldn't even finish chewing one mouthful when I'd pour in the next handful. I needed to go faster and faster to stay ahead of the disappointment and outrage that were gaining on me. I was letting myself down and I knew it. But I also knew that chocolate works fast. In a minute or two, when the sugar rush hit, I really wouldn't care!

Finally, I was full. The anxious adrenaline rush was over. I was calm and so stuffed I could barely move. I couldn't eat another bite. My stomach was starting to hurt. In less than five minutes, I'd eaten nearly half a pound of M&M's.

With a sigh, I folded the wrapper around the small amount of M&M's that were left and hid them away in the drawer with relief. As I lay back on the bed, the voice I'd been trying to run away from caught up with me.

Through my sugar haze, I could hear it complaining and criticizing me in my head. You did it again. You totally lost control. I can't believe that. How could you?

My defense sounded lame, even to me. I'm going to sleep now, I told myself. I'll wake up tomorrow with a clean slate and start my diet then. It was the lie I always used to tell myself, when I gave in. And by now I knew it wasn't the point. Starting a diet after binging was keeping me running in circles. I had to stop binging.

The feeling of defeat was overwhelming. My eyes welled up with tears. Maybe I'd never be able to have control over food. Maybe I'd have scenes like this one, over and over again for the rest of my life: one little moment of resolve, followed by a frantic five-minute binge, followed by remorse and empty promises. At this rate, I'd be overweight forever.

I thought I was forcing myself to face the facts, that I was finally being honest and seeing things as they really were. What I didn't realize was, I was making things worse. Instead of offering myself comfort and support, I'd bashed myself over the head with my failures, until I felt completely hopeless. By the time I'd finished "facing facts" I was so depressed and disgusted with myself that I couldn't take it. I was in desperate need of relief.

And sure enough, that feeling of adrenaline suddenly rose up inside me again. I found myself reaching toward the drawer to take the candy out...

What the hell was I doing? I'd just decided that this was the very thing that was ruining my life!

You're stuffed, I told myself. You couldn't eat anything else if you wanted to. You don't have to do this!

It was good advice, but I ignored myself. I unwrapped the candy, poured out a small handful, tossed it in my mouth and started chewing. Such a wave of self-hatred came over me in that moment that I burst into tears, still chewing the candy, with the candy and saliva dripping from my mouth as I cried. I was at an all-time low.

"God, if you're here," I sobbed, "I need you. I can't stop eating!"

That's all I said. Then I lay on my bed and cried like a baby.

* * *

At some point, the Sonny and Cher album finished playing. After several minutes, my tears subsided and I sat up on the edge of my bed in silence.

A tremendous feeling of peace came over me. I sat there savoring it for a moment. It was a gratifying feeling.

I felt so drained from the experience that I went to sleep for twelve hours. The next day, I wrote this in my journal:

> Had a bad day yesterday. My face is so damned bloated. Slept for twelve hours last night.

Anxious to start dieting again. Feel bad when I
stuff myself all day. Feel wonderful when I diet!
God's going to help me too. I asked him last night,
crying my eyes out. I know He heard me. After I
asked Him, a peaceful feeling came over me.

From that day on, I never once had the urge to gorge
myself. I never experienced losing control to food again. Not
once!

Oh sure, sometimes I overate at dinner parties, but I
never felt at the mercy of a compulsive urge to eat. Something
amazing happened that night to me. I was healed. I cried out to
God — really needing His help — and I got it. I didn't believe for
a second it would work, but it did. And it has, for all these years.

The strange thing is, I didn't even realize, until years
later, that I never binged again after that night. It's the kind of
thing you notice later. You see a bag of M&M's and think, Wow,
I used to gobble down a bag like that in one sitting. It's been
awhile … So gradually I noticed I'd stopped binging for good.
But I attributed it to my own self-discipline.

Then one night, years later, I was telling a girlfriend
how I used to gorge myself with food and feel completely out of
control. And suddenly it hit me: It had all changed that night,
on October 5, 1974, when I called out to God. Until then, I'd
never given God the credit. It seems so obvious, but somehow I
hadn't realized what a miracle had occurred that night.

Now I can honestly tell people that it's possible to have
compulsive behavior lifted on the spot. I know, because it
happened to me. I reached into the depths of my soul, and God
listened.

I feel so blessed to have had such an experience. The
surprising thing is, it gave me something much more important
than freedom from food. It made me recognize that there really
is a God, that there's something out there that will help us, if we
earnestly ask for help, which is beautiful to know.

* * *

I wish I could say that God made me thin that night too. But He didn't.

The compulsion was gone. I was free from that awful feeling of being out of control when it came to food. Unfortunately, when I got up that next morning I was still overweight.

Losing weight wasn't all downhill from there. I continued to struggle with dieting for years. The lack of compulsion over food made dieting easier though. When I was twenty, I got down to 156 pounds — just three pounds higher than what the weight charts said was a normal weight for my height — and maintained that weight for about a year.

By that time, though, I'd started drinking heavily, so the pounds started creeping back. A lack of compulsive eating made losing weight a lot easier, but drinking made it a lot harder. Soon I'd started gaining weight again. I wouldn't be able to get down to my normal weight again until years later, when I gave up alcohol for good.

5

Losing It

I DIDN'T REALIZE IT AT THE TIME, BUT A GOOD PART OF MY weight problem was crash dieting. Every time I lost weight in starvation mode, my body would overcompensate to get things back to normal. So I'd gain the weight back faster when I went off the diet. It was that constant cycle that leveraged me all the way up to my top weight.

If I'd wanted to gain weight, that was exactly the way to do it.

* * *

Crash diets kept me on a roller coaster for years.

Even my mom got into the game when she told me about her doctor, who had recently lost one hundred pounds on a new low-carbohydrate diet.

The high-protein/low-carb competition between fad diets was just getting started when I was in high school. If you can believe it, there was actually a time before that when only a few doctors talked about protein and carbs. Nutrisweet hadn't come out yet either. So there were no sugar-free, fat-free (nutrient-free) chocolate muffins on the grocery store shelves. If there had been, I'm sure I would've been buying boxes of those as well.

Instead, I went to see Mom's doctor. After losing one hundred pounds, he felt like a new man. So he was eager to tell me about the diet and he knew that I too wanted to lose weight as quickly as possible. But he didn't think it was a healthy diet for an adolescent. He suggested that I go on the diet for a few months to jump-start my weight loss, then switch over to a healthier, more balanced diet.

"If you limit yourself to thirty grams of carbohydrates a day," he promised, "you should lose about ten pounds a month. After you've lost twenty or thirty pounds, come back to me and we'll figure out what you should eat from there."

It sounded reasonable enough. I DID lose weight — thirty-eight pounds on the low-carb diet. On the days I dieted, I would make an attempt to follow the diet all day. But if I blew it — by eating cookies or ice cream or chips — I'd consider it a "lost" day and write it off. That gave me full permission to eat whatever I wanted the rest of the day, telling myself I'd start back on the diet the next day. I always knew there was a fifty/fifty chance that I might NOT start back on the diet the next day, but I played that game with myself for years.

What I did realize with the low-carb diet, however, was that it was pretty easy. When I did stick with it, I lost weight fairly easily. It amazes me now that I didn't jump at the chance to finally lose the weight with this relatively easy diet by sticking to it every day until I got down to 145 or so.

Instead, I was glad to know I could have the diet in my "arsenal." If ever I needed a surefire diet, I had this one — for emergencies. It gave me more permission to eat, because with this diet, I could lose weight any time.

* * *

Drugs were another way I tried to lose weight. In high school, my friend Denise started getting diet pills from her doctor. She lost a lot of weight and started looking so great, she was almost no fun to be around anymore. But my mom wouldn't take me to get the pills, so I bought them from Denise. I don't know what she told her doctor, but she must have been running short. She sold her pills to me for weeks.

They were basically amphetamines, of course. The idea was that they would make you high AND suppress your appetite. It was a double-whammy. The pills were such a rush that I didn't need the stimulus of chocolate and I wasn't hungry when it was time for lunch. To me, it seemed like the perfect solution.

I'd buy a few from Denise, then take one late in the morning. All the way through lunch, I'd be euphoric and not hungry at all. Then about five hours later, around four or five o'clock, I'd start to crash. My energy would plummet. The emotional dive would be so steep that sometimes I'd start to cry for no reason at all.

I knew it was the pills. Even though Denise never complained about this effect, I eventually stopped buying them. I loved to feel that feeling for several hours and not be hungry. But I knew they were addictive. And I worried about that. With diet pills, it seemed like the solution might create a bigger problem than it cured.

* * *

Once I started drinking coffee and smoking cigarettes, there were new stimulants available to me. With coffee and cigarettes, I didn't mind not eating. Now and then, just for a lark, I'd skip a meal and I didn't miss it.

One day, when I was working as a maid at the Ming Tree Motel, I started off early with coffee and a cigarette for breakfast. At lunch, I still wasn't all that hungry. I had another cigarette or two on my lunch break and a few more cups of coffee. I smoked two or three cigarettes an hour, killing my appetite throughout the day. When dinner rolled around, I was starting to feel a little hungry, but, by that time, I'd decided to see if I could fast for an entire day.

I did it. No problem.

Even better, when I woke up the next morning, I felt

fantastic. My stomach had shrunk from not eating the day before, so I still wasn't hungry. When I got on the scale, I grinned.

I'd lost two pounds.

Immediately, I made the decision to fast for one more day. With the coffee and cigarettes, it wasn't that hard.

When I went to bed on the second night, I was feeling pretty cocky. I had gone two days without eating and I felt great. Not many people could do that. In fact, if you mentioned it to anyone, they'd be appalled. What incredible willpower I had!

I woke up on day three and got on the scales. I'd lost five pounds in two days. It truly was amazing. I decided to fast as long as I could. Tibetan monks fast in the mountains all the time, right? Jesus fasted in the hot desert for forty days. I'd be fine.

And skinny? At this rate, I'd lose almost eighteen pounds in a week. In two weeks, I'd have lost over thirty-six pounds! My weight problem would be over for good. I went to work smiling.

By noon, I almost collapsed in one of the rooms I was cleaning.

The other maids rushed over to help me. When I told them I'd been fasting for two and a half days, they told me they were going to feed me, that I had to eat or I'd pass out.

I couldn't eat much at lunch but by the next day, I was eating normally again and I quickly gained the several pounds of water weight I'd lost by sending my body into shock.

After that experience, I never tried fasting again, though I did skip meals. I read a breathless article in a magazine about how five different TV actresses maintained their figures. One of them revealed her secret: She never ate after noontime. So I thought I'd try it.

I allowed myself to eat anything I wanted in the morning as long as I stopped by noon. It was practically a fast, since it meant not eating for about twenty hours.

But that's a long time to go without food. And there's nothing pleasant about going to sleep on an empty stomach — especially when you've been hungry for hours. Once in awhile I could finish out the day without eating, but those days were few and far between.

I blamed myself for not getting better results. But if I'd known then what I know now, I would've realized that fasting for twenty hours would've lowered my metabolism so much that it would have gradually become much harder for me to lose weight and much, much easier to gain it back.

*   *   *

Like most people, I was eager to believe what the experts said — whether they were beautiful actresses who were clearly doing something right or doctors promoting their diet books or weight loss treatment centers with a fancy new treatment that everyone was raving about.

When Slim Wrap opened a treatment center in my town for a short while, a lot of people signed up. They promised they could take several inches off your body in a few hours. One wrap was supposed to be like twenty hours of exercising. Their brochures had lots of testimonials from people who claimed to have lost a dress size after a single Slim Wrap treatment. It was all the rage.

So my friend Denise and I tried it out. We were each led into our own private changing room and told to take off all of our clothes. When you're overweight and self-conscious about your body, the last thing you want to do is take off your clothes in public. I didn't even want the employee to see me naked, a total stranger who looked like she'd never been overweight a day in her life. But I'd try anything to lose weight.

The total stranger smiled politely as she wrapped her tape measure around me, jotting down measurements from my entire body. Then I stood in a special alcove while she dipped long cloths into the Slim Wrap solution, then wrapped them around me snugly, like Ace bandages around a sprained ankle.

The only parts of my body left unwrapped were my head, my hands and my feet. I wondered about the wisdom of this. Were my head, my hands and my feet any less fat than any other part of me? Shouldn't she wrap me up like a mummy, just to be sure?

I had plenty of time to think about it. After the stranger wound the dripping cloths around me, she led me to a cot. "Lay here and rest," she said sweetly. "Clear your mind and just let the solution do its work…"

After about two hours, she came back and led me to the changing room again. One by one, she peeled the wet cloths off. Then she measured me again.

"Oh, this is very good," she said. "You've lost an inch from your hips and two inches from your waist. Your left thigh is half an inch smaller than it was two hours ago and…" She paused, wrapping the measuring tape around my right thigh. "And so is your right thigh."

She played her part well, but I found it completely unconvincing. I was looking in the mirror as she was measuring. I wanted to see the changes a lot more than she did, but I didn't notice anything different.

Two hours of my life, lying in wet cloths covered with goo, for absolutely no reason at all. And that wasn't as far as I would go to lose weight. I'd go further…

* * *

When the opportunity arose, I was actually shot up with urine from pregnant women. And I paid for the privilege.

There was a place in town called the Weight Control Clinic. One of their latest, most effective techniques was to collect urine from women who were pregnant and resell it to women who were overweight. For thirty dollars a week, you could come into the clinic, sit down in a plastic chair and have a nurse inject you with urine.

To make the idea more appealing, the marketing materials promised you could eat anything you wanted afterward. In fact, the more you ate, the better.

"For the urine to take effect," the nurses advised, "you must eat enough so the fat cells in your body are mobilized right away. That starts the process of losing weight."

"You mean stuff myself?" I asked.

The nurse nodded. "For two days."

Since the urine injections were after my experience of calling out to God I hadn't stuffed myself in years. The experience hadn't made me miraculously lose weight overnight, but it had stopped my compulsive eating, and I didn't like the idea of stuffing myself because of the urine. But I did follow directions and ate whatever and whenever I wanted for two days.

As I understand it, there is little to no evidence that the urine of pregnant women has any effect on weight loss in other people, even if you inject it directly into their bodies. It was just one more thing I was willing to believe, if there was even a chance that it would help me lose weight.

6

Firsts

WHEN YOU GRADUATE HIGH SCHOOL AND WALK OUT INTO the world as an adult, you end up doing a lot of things for the first time.

My time after high school was filled with firsts. The first time I went to college. The first time I was thin. The first time I took a drink. The first time I fell in love with an older man.

For better or worse, some of these things turn into habits that set the pattern for the rest of your life. Others are more fleeting. You explore them for awhile and then discard them later. Sometimes ten or twenty years later, if you're like me.

After high school, all I really cared about were my boyfriends, my drinking and my weight problem. For longer than I like to remember, those three things were the only things that mattered.

It had all started with my first boyfriend. I met him when I was sixteen and we dated off and on for three years. During that time, nothing in my life was more important to me than Ron. It's not that he was such a great boyfriend, it's just that I thought he was the best I could do. I weighed 210 pounds and, even though he didn't like it, he kept dating me, so I put up with a lot from him.

In the beginning, it had been very romantic. He invited me to his apartment, then he pulled out a Stevie Wonder album. The first song was fast and Ron started dancing around the living room, trying to impress me. It worked! He was a great dancer. And it was sexy, watching him dance. I was incredibly attracted to him.

The next song was a slow dance, love song. Ron slowly walked over to me, smiling, then pushed me backward onto the couch and lay down on top of me. I had never kissed a guy before, not the way he kissed me. After that first kiss, I felt connected to him and so in love. I had never experienced feelings of love like that for a man before.

Once we made love, those feelings were heightened. For a long time, he was the only man I'd ever had sex with. It made me feel such a bond with him that I couldn't break up with him for three years, even when I discovered he wasn't being faithful.

He'd even use me for transportation when he went out to spend the night with other girls because he didn't have a car. I was so young and in love that I stayed with him anyway. He constantly told me he loved me to keep me hooked. Things weren't right and I knew it. But I also knew he genuinely liked me. And I was still overweight. So I honestly thought that having a loser like Ron was the best I could do.

I told myself that, if I'd only lose weight, he'd really fall in love with me and stop fooling around. So I kept trying, but it felt hopeless. I'd lose a little weight, then gain it back. Once I got down to 180 pounds, Ron's interest in me did pick up but that didn't change his interest in other women.

By the time we broke up, I'd established the first part of the pattern that was going to govern my life for years. All I thought about was my boyfriend and my weight. Then, before I knew it, I was going to shift that pattern just a bit to add to a series of boyfriends a whole new fascination: drinking.

* * *

When I first started drinking, I was in Hawaii with my friend Carol. We were both nineteen years old. It was the first time either of us had been to Hawaii. Drinking seemed like the natural thing to do.

My father had paid for my plane fare. He said it was time for me to move away from Santa Barbara and explore other places. So this was his way of "pushing me out of the nest." He offered to pay for me to go to the University of Hawaii while I was there, too, but I didn't go.

I'd started Santa Barbara City College, but I couldn't get into it. Initially, I'd signed up for four classes, but I didn't make any effort to pass. So I ended up dropping two of them before my low grades spoiled my record. The next semester, I'd tried again — starting off with three classes. But I'd soon dropped all of them. I thought college was a good idea. I just didn't care.

The only good part was I met Carol in Algebra. We started talking about how cool it would be to live in Hawaii and one thing led to another. Before we knew it, we were sharing a three-hundred-dollar-a-month furnished studio in Waikiki.

Both of us found jobs during the day to cover our expenses. At night, we joined the locals and the tourists at the island bars and nightclubs along the beach. The drinking age was eighteen in Hawaii and I was ecstatic that I could drink.

When we first started going to the nightclubs, Carol and I would get carded. We thought that was cool! Being able to actually be in a nightclub was new to Carol and me and we could hardly believe they were letting us in at all. Every night felt like a party. It suited me perfectly, even when I was sober. But once I started drinking, I thought I'd died and gone to heaven. Alcohol made me feel happy and carefree and I quickly found a favorite drink: a Mai Tai.

I'd always loved the rush of eating a pint of vanilla ice cream or a big bag of chocolate chip cookies. And I soon discovered that alcohol was even better. A warm, pleasurable feeling seeped into me after I'd had a few drinks. Suddenly, I felt confident and friendly. I'd say hello to everybody and try to make them smile. I felt great and I wanted them to feel great too.

The food I'd gotten high on when I was a kid, back in high school, had never made me feel gregarious. I'd feel better, but I'd stay in my room in my nightgown, watching TV or pretending I was Cher. With alcohol, I didn't have to pretend. I was Cher!

Suddenly, I was the life of the party. I talked to everybody and I loved to dance. When I first walked into a club, I was friendly, but I would never have asked a stranger if he wanted to dance. Two or three drinks later, I felt so confident that I didn't even wait for guys to ask me to dance. Whenever I heard a song I liked, I'd just get up and start walking to the dance floor. On the way, I'd ask any guy I saw to dance. Drinking a lot gave me courage and boldness.

Carol and I were two single, nineteen-year-old girls in the Land of Paradise. What was not to love?

* * *

On the flight over, Carol and I made a solemn pact. We were going to lose weight in Hawaii. We spent half the flight talking about the bikinis we were going to wear — and look fabulous in — on the beach. Those drinks with tiny little umbrellas were going to fall out of men's hands, as they stood drooling, when we strolled by.

Carol was about fifteen pounds overweight; I was about twenty-five pounds overweight. We decided that paradise was just what we needed to lose weight.

And it worked! We never actually saw men drop their drinks because of us. But we never had a shortage of attention either.

Part of the reason for our success was that it was hot and humid from the time we got off the plane the first day. For three days, we drank so much water that we were bloated, until our systems got used to the hot weather. Between the heat and the water, neither one of us was hungry. So we ate a lot less.

And we walked all around Waikiki — probably several miles every day. We'd get up at 4:00 A.M. and go to the twenty-four-hour coffee shop to have several cups of coffee. Then we'd go for an hour's walk. After ten in the morning, it got uncomfortably hot, the tourists came out and everything was so crowded, it wasn't much fun. But in the early morning, we could have Waikiki all to ourselves and we loved it.

It was a painless way to lose weight. We hardly noticed it was happening. But, before we knew it, our clothes were loose and we did look pretty great in our bikinis.

I kept the weight off for awhile, but I gradually gained those fourteen pounds back. By the time I was twenty-four, I'd crept back up to 185.

Unfortunately, I hadn't made exercise a new habit. I'd made drinking a habit instead. And I wouldn't get back down to a good weight for me until I gave up drinking. From the time I was twenty to thirty-one years old, my weight fluctuated between 165 and 185 pounds.

Back in the states, I didn't exercise. I barely even walked. Like most Californians, I drove everywhere — even if the store I was going to was a few blocks away. I liked the idea of being thin. Hardly a day went by when I didn't think about it. But I continued to avoid exercise, eat high-fat/high-calorie foods and drink as much alcohol as I reasonably could.

Still, I did make efforts. For awhile, I started drinking gin and tonics because I heard that gin had zero carbohydrates. I was pretty happy with this plan. And then I found some sugar-free tonic water, which meant I could make drinks with ZERO carbohydrates! I was thrilled. That meant I could drink and stay on my high-protein/low-carb diet at the same time.

The only trouble was, when I was buzzed — much less drunk — I couldn't stomach high-protein foods. I needed foods with major carbs, like chips and bread and pizza. If I drank three or four gin and tonics, then tried to eat my cottage cheese and hamburger patty, my stomach would revolt. I'd feel like throwing up. And that would ruin my high.

"Okay," I finally told myself one day. "You're going to have to face it. You can't go on a high-protein/low-carb diet until later ... when you stop drinking for awhile."

It was disappointing. But somehow I found a way to accept it.

* * *

Years went by before I made it back down to the 156 I weighed on that first trip to Hawaii. But I never forgot the feeling. It had been the first time in my life I'd felt thin. I'd gotten a taste of what it would feel like to have confidence in my body.

It was a whole new experience to cross a dance floor without worrying that all the men were thinking I was fat. Gradually, I began to realize that they were now thinking how great I looked and wondering if they could have the next dance!

Before too long, I found I'd fallen in love with one of them.

Isaiah was a twenty-eight-year-old contractor I'd met in Honolulu. He lavished attention on me. He'd work all day, then come by my studio around 8:00 P.M. to take me out for drinks at the clubs. Sometimes he would get us a hotel room and spend the night with me. It was exciting — being nineteen years old and having an older man being interested enough to buy me dinner, drinks and a room. Sometimes I felt like a kept woman and I liked it.

Since I always got drunk when we went out, I would also be hung over the next day. It was sweet to wake up in the morning with a splitting headache and find a note from Isaiah, saying something like, "Good morning, sweetheart. Buy some breakfast when you wake up." He knew I was on a tight budget,

66

so he'd leave ten dollars for breakfast on the table next to the note. Isaiah was attentive and caring. I really enjoyed getting his attention. Before long, I'd opened my heart and fallen in love.

But as the weeks went by, things began to change. Often, I'd sit smoking cigarette after cigarette waiting for Isaiah to show up for our date. If he called, he'd always have an excuse about why he couldn't come by that night. Sometimes, he wouldn't call at all. Then the next day, he'd make up a reason about why he hadn't been there and hadn't even bothered to pick up the phone.

Of course, I really grilled him. ("Are you telling me the truth?" I'd say. "Oh, yes! I love you so much. I have no reason to lie!" he'd swear.) But because I loved him, I stupidly believed his excuses … for awhile.

"He's pulling the wool over your eyes, you know," Carol warned me. "You just don't want to see it."

What I didn't see and couldn't see was that Isaiah had a wife and two young kids he'd never told me about. When I found out, I was devastated. I thought about breaking it off on the spot, but Isaiah assured me that I was the one he truly loved and he would rather leave his wife and kids than lose me.

Like millions of women before me, I bought it. But before long, I started putting things together. Here was a man who had lied to me about having a family. Why should I think for a minute that he would tell me the truth about leaving his family?

It's undoubtedly a difficult thing to tell your wife you want a divorce, but it doesn't take a lot of time to say, "I'm leaving you." After three months of broken promises, I realized Isaiah had no intention of saying it.

I called my mom in California and asked her to buy me a plane ticket home. She was resistant at first.

"You're leaving already?"

"Yes, Mom. Please. I've got to. I'll pay you back as soon as I start working again."

"Why don't you stay a little longer, then see how you feel?" she coaxed, thinking I just needed encouragement. "You're giving up too soon."

"No, Mom," I insisted. "I have to come home!" And then I pulled out my best bargaining chip. "If you'll buy me the ticket, I'll finish college when I get back."

I knew she couldn't say no to that. And she didn't. She bought me the ticket for the next day.

Isaiah drove me silently to the airport in Honolulu. I was on the verge of tears. When I was ready to board the plane, we hugged and I cried.

"It's not goodbye," he said, trying not to get emotional. "I'll book a flight and come over to see you next week, okay? I don't want to lose you!"

A little flutter of hope skipped across my heart. Maybe he was serious about leaving his wife after all...

Over the next several weeks, Isaiah called many times. I'd get so excited because he'd say, "I'm going to buy a plane ticket and be there tomorrow," and then I wouldn't hear from him for days. He always had an excuse. And he never came.

After a few months, I took an honest look at what I was doing. I was waiting for a lying, cheating married man!

As soon as I saw it clearly, something switched inside me. I realized he had never really planned to come to California. It was all talk. The next time he called, I felt so different — so strong.

"You're never going to come," I told him, flatly, as if stating the obvious.

"Linda, how can you say that? Of course I'm going to come. Things have just been up in the air the past few weeks and I haven't been able to make it. But you know I miss you."

"If you miss me, come tomorrow."

"I would love to, but I can't. I promise I'll be over soon!"

This time, the lie was so blatant, it didn't hook me anymore. Instead, I realized I didn't want him to come. Just days before, I'd been wishing with all my heart that Isaiah would come. Now, here I was really hoping that he would NOT come! It was such an amazing change of heart that it astonished me.

A feeling of strength came over me. I'd spent months crying over this man, believing his promises, waiting by the phone. He'd lied to me — and to his family — over and over again. But I had come through that whole ordeal — by myself and on my own. I couldn't help but smile.

And then it occurred to me. What if, after all this time, he did actually jump on a plane and fly over? That would ruin everything! So I made up a lie of my own. "The thing is, Isaiah, there's this guy I've been seeing that I really like a lot…"

As I explained about my fictional romance, it was quiet on the other end of the line. Something between us had shifted for good. "Just remember, Linda," Isaiah said softly, "I'll always love you."

For a split second, I wondered. Was he lying or telling the truth?

To my amazement, I wasn't very interested in knowing anymore. It was as if all of my feelings and emotions for Isaiah had vanished in an instant.

There was no new romance in my life at the moment. But I might come across one any minute now. It was time to move on.

"Okay, Isaiah. Bye. I gotta go."

7

Mixers

OVER THE NEXT SEVERAL YEARS, I MIXED MEN AND ALCOHOL together indiscriminately. After my experiences in Hawaii, I was determined to stop dating losers like Ron and Isaiah, but before long I was drinking so heavily that any man who wasn't a loser would have known enough to keep his distance. And to tell you the truth, drunk as I was most of the time, I didn't always know the difference.

For awhile I went out with a very gentle guy named Allan, who was several years older than I was. I'd met him through Ron years before, and Allan had been so taken with me that he kept asking me out and finally I agreed.

Before long we were living together. With my fear of being alone, it was comforting to have someone to come home to, but it didn't change my feelings for Allan. Even when we were having sex together and spending every night in the same bed, I made it clear that the relationship wasn't exclusive and it wasn't serious. What teenagers call "friends with benefits" today, we just called "friends" in the eighties. Since Allan adored me, he didn't mind what we called it, as long as he could be with me. He didn't even mind that I weighed 185 pounds at the time. He generously offered to help me lose weight, if I'd let him. But I never did.

Being friends allowed me to keep going out and picking up other men, if I felt like it. So I went out to meet people for drinks on a regular basis and almost always came home raging drunk. I'd yell at Allan, call him names and tell him I wasn't happy staying with him because he wasn't my boyfriend.

"You don't mean that," Allan would say, kindly, reaching out to wrap me in his arms.

But his gentleness was wasted on me when I was drunk. I'd push my way past him. "Oh yes, I do mean it!" I'd scream. "I'm sick of living here with you! I've had it! I'm moving out first thing in the morning!" And then I'd pass out on the bed.

I realized I was mistreating Allan, but I was so frustrated to be in an unfulfilled relationship that I took it out on him without remorse. I blamed him for my unhappiness. If he'd been a better, more interesting guy, I would've loved spending time with him. But he just didn't measure up. Somehow I always thought I deserved a better guy. But every guy I dated had serious flaws, in my eyes. So a lot of my relationships ended up like this.

As much as he adored me, this kind of behavior eventually wore thin with Allan. He started by insisting that I not drink while I was living with him. When that didn't work, he asked me to leave.

"I don't know who you are anymore," he told me, sadly. "You've changed — into someone who scares me."

* * *

I found a one-bedroom apartment and lived there for about six months. Just as I'd expected, it was easy to meet new guys at the bars and, if I played my cards right, I was never in too much danger of being alone — or even driving drunk.

If I was too drunk to drive and I met someone I liked, whom I felt I could trust, I'd let him take me home. If I wasn't drunk enough to fall immediately asleep as soon as I hit the bed, I'd invite him in to keep me company. I didn't worry about it too much, because I thought of myself as a good judge of character. When I'm sober, it's true. I am a good judge of character. But when I'm drunk, that skill, like everything else, tends to blur.

One night, I went to a bar to meet my friend Star. I was still only twenty, but we knew the bouncer and he always let us in. While I was getting my beer, I noticed a young guy watching me from across the room. He was one of the most handsome guys who'd ever shown an interest in me. I was thrilled. Coyly lowering my eyes, I lifted my drink to my lips and took a sip, then glanced over discreetly to see if he was still looking at me, but he was gone. My heart dropped for an instant, and then I realized he was making his way over to me. Our eyes met as he approached. I couldn't help but smile.

"Would you like to dance?" he said, leaning close to whisper in my ear.

We danced a few sets together, and then went to join Star at a table nearby. She had met someone too. I loved the image: two attractive couples, laughing and sharing drinks at a table in a bar. I'd looked on with envy to this kind of scene many times, but had never been a part of that scene myself. In fact, I'd never felt like a couple with an attractive man who wasn't a loser. I wanted Jim to fall in love with me. Then I could have this experience all the time. Jim was a pharmacist — a respectable job! He'd danced well and put his arm around me as he escorted me to the table. It was perfect. I looked around at the other people in the room to see if we were being watched.

When Jim took me home that night, I gave him my phone number. He explained that he had to go out of town so I might not hear from him all week, but he'd love to take me out for dinner and drinks the following Friday night, if I wanted to go. Of course, I said yes. And I fantasized all week about Jim.

When he picked me up that Friday, he casually asked where I'd like to go for drinks. Being only twenty years old, there were only a few places I knew I could probably get into. I was excited about the date and I didn't want the evening to go badly because I was underage. But I didn't want to make an issue of my age with Jim either. So, crossing my fingers, I suggested a few bars nearby.

Jim dismissed those choices and said he'd take me to a better place — a bar close to the beach that had great Margaritas. When we got there, we found a table, and then Jim went to the bar and ordered a half liter of Margaritas. The waiter delivered it to our table. No questions about my age at all. Even before I was twenty-one, I was learning how to get my drinks delivered to me, any time, anywhere. A half liter of Margaritas meant about 1.5 drinks for each of us, but I noticed I got two drinks out of it, while Jim drank one. Then he ordered another half liter.

After we'd had some great hors d'oeuvres, Jim asked me where I wanted to go for dinner. By that time, I'd had four Margaritas and wasn't hungry in the least. In fact, I was drunk.

"But I'm full now from eating the hors d'oeuvres!" I said, speaking very carefully. "Let's just have a few more Margaritas."

"Hors d'oeuvres aren't dinner," Jim said. "I want to take you to a nice dinner. Where shall we go?"

"I really can't eat anything else," I insisted. "That's all for me."

Jim smiled and took my hand. "Well, then, we could always go back to your place…"

As soon as we walked into my apartment, Jim started kissing me. I was very drunk, but also very turned on! We never even made it to the bedroom. In moments, we were on the living room floor. The room was starting to heat up. Our clothes were starting to come off. We kissed for several minutes. Then suddenly Jim stopped. He pulled away and stood up. I didn't know what was happening.

"I'm sorry, Linda," he said. "I have to stop."

"Why? Why do you have to stop?" I winced, sitting up on the floor.

"You're really beautiful, Linda, but I shouldn't have started anything with you. I have a fiancée and we're getting married next year. If it wasn't for that, I'd be very interested in dating you. I'm sorry."

Without another word, he stood up, put his shirt back on, turned and walked out the door. I wanted to cry. I had been so excited about this guy all week. I made myself a couple of gin and tonics and sat on the couch playing music, smoking cigarettes and crying.

But I wasn't entirely miserable. After all, Jim had said that I was beautiful and that he'd be interested in me if he didn't have a fiancée. A handsome man with a respectable job wanted to go out with me. That wasn't all bad.

* * *

Once I got over the rejection, the very idea that such a good-looking man had been attracted to me — would've been dating me, if it hadn't been for some pre-existing woman — cheered me up for weeks. We really could have been that perfect couple at the table, laughing and having a good time, if he'd been free. It was a happy thought.

Skip was not nearly as good looking. He was on the short side for a guy. At 5'9" tall, I towered over him by three inches. He was stocky, with long, wavy red hair. I didn't find him attractive at all, but he paid a lot of attention to me and I liked that.

We attended Santa Barbara City College together. On the breaks, we hung out a lot in the cafeteria, drinking coffee, smoking cigarettes and skipping classes. It was good to have a friend to hang around with, except that Skip was always hitting on me. I told him repeatedly I wasn't interested in him that way, but he kept at it.

One day, he unexpectedly dropped into a chair next to me at the cafeteria. "Let's go out Friday night," he said.

"No, Skip. I told you. We're not going out."

Before I knew what was happening, he raised a felt-tipped pen and made an "X" on my cheek. It was over so fast, I didn't know what was happening.

"I officially cross you off my list," he said sternly and walked away.

Students at the nearby tables snickered. I felt like a fool. It was such a bizarre thing to do that, if I'd had any sense, I would've cut him off completely after that. A few years later, Skip lost his temper and attacked a bus driver with a baseball bat. He ended up going to prison for years. When we were in school together, I didn't know he was capable of going so far. I only knew he was a loser. But I didn't cut him off. He was one of the few people who would go out to bars drinking with me, so, as strange as he was, I couldn't afford to lose him — at least not during the week.

On weekends, I could meet men easily if I went out drinking and dancing with a girlfriend. At some of the clubs, there were a lot of Arab guys. With their dark, swarthy looks, they were appealing and they often treated women with a graciousness that was less common in the local men. Sometimes I'd sit and talk with one or two of the Arab men, then get so drunk I'd end up going home with one of them. As far as I could remember, I usually had a good time — at least, that was my impression.

Either way, Skip didn't fit into my weekend plans. If we went out drinking together at all, it was during the week. Since he didn't have a car, we always took mine.

One Wednesday night, Skip and I went to one of the clubs where I'd meet my Arab friends on the weekends. When we sat down at our table, I didn't expect to see anyone I knew there on a weeknight. We sat, drinking wine and enjoying the music for about an hour, when Fahad, one of the Arab men I had a crush on, came in with another man. They sat at a corner table across the room. I waved to Fahad, then went over to say hi. "I'll be right back," I told Skip.

When I came back to our table, Skip was angry. "Look, you're here with me. I don't appreciate you talking to other guys." We'd both had a lot to drink by this time, so the more Skip talked, the louder he got.

"Shhh!" I said. "You're making a scene. People are watching us." By "people," I meant Fahad and his friend.

Skip looked over and saw them looking our way. "Then give me a kiss," he said, putting his arm around me and trying to pull me closer.

"Don't be disgusting!" I said, getting up from the table in a huff. "We're leaving! NOW! I'm taking you home."

Skip was suitably humiliated. Not only was I publicly pushing him away when he was trying to kiss me, but I was driving him home as well. He got up from the table, looking dejected.

I smiled across the room at Fahad, indicating that we had to leave. He motioned for me to come over to his table. I started walking over to Fahad, trying to maintain and not stumble. We'd gone out a few times and I really liked this guy. I was hoping he was calling me over to his table so he could ask me out again.

When I got there, he said, "I'm sorry, Linda, but I just want you to know we can't go out together anymore. In my country, we don't get in the way if a woman is seeing another man."

"Oh, no!" I cried. "Skip is just a friend. I don't even like him. Please, believe me. Don't even think about it. He's nothing." I stood grinning, trying not to wobble. "We can still go out. I really like you a lot!"

"I'm sorry, Linda. I hope you will be happy together."

I could see Fahad had made up his mind. There was nothing I could do. I turned and walked back to Skip. When I saw him, I felt absolute disgust.

Skip was standing there, waiting for me, a look of pure drunkenness on his face. "Did I get your boyfriend mad? Good!"

I picked up my purse and walked out the door. I was in no condition to drive, but Skip's house was ten miles away — too expensive to take a taxi. So I drove with one eye closed and one eye opened, trying to focus. I drove slowly along the back roads, still thinking about Fahad and cursing Skip under my breath.

It was almost midnight when we passed a twenty-four-hour diner near Skip's house. I was drunk and hungry. "Let's get something to eat," I told Skip. Fahad and I had been to this place after hours. There weren't many places opened late and I knew he liked this one.

As luck would have it, as soon as Skip and I ordered, Fahad and his friend came strolling in.

"Is that that same guy?" Skip snarled, as Fahad walked by. "You're with me tonight. Don't forget it!"

"Shut up!" I snapped, getting up from the table. Steadying myself on the backs of the booths, as I crossed the diner, I made my way over to Fahad. I pleaded with him to forget about Skip and explained again, slurring my words hopelessly, that we weren't together. We were just friends.

"Linda, please go," Fahad said, losing patience. "Don't talk to me anymore."

Drunk and devastated, I walked straight out of the diner and got in my car. By the time Skip realized what was happening and ran outside, I was pulling out of the parking lot. He rushed at the car and slammed his palm down on the hood.

"YOU RUINED EVERYTHING," I screamed, slamming on the brakes.

"You can't leave me here. I have no way to get home," Skip said.

Reluctantly, I opened the door and let him in. As soon as he was in the car, I started crying. "When I drop you off, I never want to see you again. You ruined it for me and Fahad."

"You're a slut," Skip yelled. "All this time, you've just been using me to have somebody to go to bars with. Well, I've had it. I'm not going to associate with sluts any longer."

I reached across the car and slapped him, hard. Skip smiled, loving the attention.

We kept yelling the entire way to his house. In between I slapped him as much as I could, but he started dodging me so I didn't always hit his face. When I came to a stop sign a few blocks from his home he jumped out. I floored it and drove right past him, back to the freeway.

As soon as I was alone I started wailing. The night had been a total disaster. I reached for a cigarette and noticed my hands were shaking as I lit it up. Then I turned slowly onto the onramp.

A red flashing light showed up in my rearview mirror. It was the highway patrol. When I pulled over, one of the highway patrolmen came up to my window and said, "We've been watching you for a few blocks and we can see that you're upset. Have you been drinking?"

"No, I just had a fight with my boyfriend," I said, crying even harder. Even in my drunken stupor, I felt proud of what an ingenious thing that was to say.

"Okay, Miss," the patrolman said, sympathetically. "We'll watch you pull away. Take it easy now."

I sniffed loudly, dabbing my tears. "Okay. Thank you, Officer," I whimpered. And as I pulled away, I added, "Sucker!"

8

Fooling Some of the People, Some of the Time

CONSIDERING HOW MUCH I WAS DRINKING IN THOSE DAYS, I'm amazed by how often I fooled people. Police officers would let me off with a warning. Bartenders would pour me another round. Even my closest friends didn't seem to realize, at first, that I was drinking myself into oblivion every chance I got.

By the time I dropped out of college, I was drinking so heavily that I didn't have the remotest idea what was going on in most of my classes. After finishing the two-year requirement at Santa Barbara City College, I'd spent a year at Cal State Northridge, a four-year college, but then I let it go. I told my dad I needed time to "decide what I wanted to do with my life." But I knew what I wanted to do. I wanted to drink — for the foreseeable future, or as long as I could get away with it.

My best friend, Elizabeth, was the opposite. She'd finished her four-year college degree in three and a half years. She'd gone to a private, Catholic college on full scholarship and devoted all of her attention to reaching her goals. So when Elizabeth sent me the invitation to her college graduation, it felt like a rebuke. I could practically see the words emblazoned on her invitation: "Elizabeth is graduating. What's your problem?"

The graduation ceremony was out of town, in Los Angeles, and I didn't want to go. I felt embarrassed. I'd finished two years of city college and got my A.A. degree (even though it took me five years to get it), so I wasn't that far behind. But Elizabeth had graduated early. She was building a happy, stable relationship with Robert. Elizabeth had her whole life together.

79

And whether anyone else realized it or not, my life was falling apart.

My sister Julie went to the ceremony with me. I could put on a good show and fool everybody else, but I needed Julie by my side for moral support. The ceremony itself wasn't so bad, but I felt a stab of jealousy when I saw Elizabeth with Robert. When she came out into the courtyard at the college in her graduation robe, he walked toward her smiling and gave her flowers. When they kissed, they looked happy together. I'd never had anyone in my life that I could love like that.

Their happiness depressed me. I needed a drink.

We'd all been invited to go to a restaurant for lunch with Elizabeth's parents, relatives and friends after the ceremony. Julie and I drove over there quickly, so we could have a glass of wine first. I needed it to make it through the lunch, pretend I was having a good time and to be able to show my enthusiasm for the new graduate.

When everyone arrived, they all started eating and I had a few more glasses of wine. Everyone was ordering alcohol. No one noticed that I was ordering more than the rest of them. It was such a lucky break to be able to order all of the wine I wanted without anyone paying attention to me, counting my drinks, or asking rudely, "Don't you think you've had enough?"

The whole time, Elizabeth and Robert kept hugging one another and whispering together, gazing into each other's eyes. And I kept ordering another drink.

Before long, Elizabeth hit her glass with her spoon to get everyone's attention. "Thank you all for coming," she said, standing. "This is a special day for me for two reasons: First, because I've just graduated from college. And second," here she smiled and sat on Robert's lap, "because I am announcing here — to my friends and family — that Robert and I are getting married in October!"

It was a jubilant moment. Everyone clapped and

cheered. There was excitement and joy in the air for the happy couple. We were all having such a good time. I felt a sense of anxiety permeating my entire body. I certainly clapped and smiled. I couldn't avoid doing that. But I kept thinking how it should have been me being happy, getting married — having two special reasons to celebrate.

Envy, that's what I was feeling. Not pride or joy or good wishes for my best friend, but envy. I knew I shouldn't feel it, but I did. I hated to admit it, but the truth was, I wasn't happy for Elizabeth.

By the time Julie and I left, I was pretty buzzed from the numerous glasses of wine I'd imbibed. But it hadn't been nearly enough. "You want to stop at that liquor store by the house and get some wine when we get back to Santa Barbara?" I asked.

Julie took one look at me, saw the desperate expression in my eyes and instantly agreed. It took one and a half hours to drive back home that Saturday afternoon. It was clear I shouldn't have been driving, because I was very drunk.

I always treated the freeway like a Free Zone when I was drunk. I told myself it was easier to drive drunk on the freeway because it was well-lit and didn't have cross-streets with stop signs that could sneak up on you. It didn't have any convenient buildings or bushes for the highway patrol to hide behind either! I felt certain the cops would never notice me amid the mass of cars on the freeway at any given time. Drunk as I was sometimes, I'm sure my weaving was conspicuous, even if I did manage to stay in my own lane. But I liked to think otherwise.

On the way home, I told Julie about my being jealous of Elizabeth. It was like "getting it out of my system" in a therapy session. I felt almost cured. I was always open and honest with Julie. She was my drinking companion and I kept no secrets from her, even though what I shared with her was embarrassing at times. But once we started drinking again, the jealousy came back in full force.

As soon as we got home, I downed another glass of wine with Julie, telling her how envious I was of Elizabeth and Robert and how I never thought I could be as happy as they were.

Since I was drunk, I didn't pretend to feel happy for them. I sincerely hoped Elizabeth and Robert wouldn't get married. I tried to cheer myself up by thinking of all the things that could go wrong. They could get into a big fight and call off the wedding — after all, they'd only been dating for four months or so. That kind of thing happened all the time.

"And, you know what else?" I told Julie, nodding my head as if this were the real corker. "Elizabeth is actually the 'older woman.' That's never going to work!"

"She's older than he is?" Julie asked groggily, taking another swig of wine.

"Oh yeah," I smirked. "Robert's twenty-three. Elizabeth is twenty-SIX!"

Julie just stared at me for a minute, like she was trying to put the pieces together. I found it incredibly annoying.

I continued, "So, obviously...he could wake up one morning and realize he's much too young to get married. He'd have to give up dating. He'd be stuck with her for the rest of his life! She may be ready for that kind of thing, but he's just a kid." October was a long way off. There was plenty of time for a disaster.

"I have history with Elizabeth," I needlessly explained to Julie. "I haven't seen her much lately, maybe twice a year, but that's just because she doesn't like to drink, so there's no point. But we go way back." I poured myself another glass of wine. "If she marries Robert, I'll never see her. I won't have a best friend anymore."

I'd always thought I was Elizabeth's best friend. So it came as a surprise to me when Elizabeth didn't choose me as her maid of honor.

I was upset at first, but then I realized I was happy not to be chosen maid of honor because of all the work it would be for me. It would also mean I'd have to spend a lot more time acting as if I were happy about Elizabeth getting married. So being a bridesmaid instead was a blessing.

* * *

As usual, the real focal point of the rehearsal dinner and the wedding itself was the drinking. At the dinner before the wedding rehearsal, everything was free, including drinks, so there was definitely an upside to Elizabeth getting married. I had a few Bloody Marys and a few Tequila Sunrises, and then ate a light dinner. I tried my best to look pleasant while I sat at the table, toasting appropriately and getting buzzed.

At the wedding rehearsal the next day, we were supposed to meet at the church at 7:00 P.M. I dreaded having to go and act happy again for Elizabeth. I asked Julie to go out with me for a few drinks first, then I could drop her off at home before going to the rehearsal. We went to a nice restaurant in town that I knew served huge glasses of wine. I was going to need lots of alcohol to make it through the hours of cheer and joy at that rehearsal.

A half-hour before I had to go, I'd already had two huge glasses of wine, but felt I could use one more. I guzzled it down in about twenty minutes. I thought I was slightly buzzed, but the wine really hit me when I stood up. I was drunk and giddy. We were laughing all the way to the car.

By the time I dropped Julie off at home, I was feeling GOOD and ready to take on the wedding rehearsal. Maybe the night wouldn't be so bad. I hated having to be there at all. And I wasn't used to doing things that I didn't want to.

When I walked into the church, the rehearsal was already underway.

"You're late," Elizabeth's mother whispered to me in the lobby. "We started fifteen minutes ago!"

From the front of the church, Elizabeth turned to see

that I'd come in. I gave her a wave. She looked a little miffed.

"I've got to go to the bathroom!" I said, urgently, to Elizabeth's mother.

"Right now?" she asked.

"YES!" After all that wine, I needed relief.

"The bathroom's outside," she said.

Almost as soon as I'd arrived, I turned around and went back outside. Elizabeth gave me a look, but I didn't care. Let her wait for me.

I walked over to the bathroom doors on the side of the building, but they were locked. That's when I saw a nun, in a long, black habit, strolling by.

"Oh, Sister," I called, giggling slightly. Since I'm not Catholic, the whole Father-Sister-Mother-Child thing had always struck me as quirky and amusing. When I was drunk, it seemed even funnier.

"Yes, dear," she said, coming toward me earnestly.

I snickered just a bit. "I have to go to the bathroom — it's an emergency — and this door is locked," I explained. "Is there a bathroom anywhere I can use?"

The rectory was right behind the church. The nun took me over there and knocked on the door. "This is very unusual," she said. "But I'm sure Father Mark and Father James will allow you to come in and use the bathroom — since it's an emergency."

When a priest opened the door, she explained my predicament. I couldn't tell whether she knew how drunk I was or not. If she was aware of it, she didn't let on. I was on the lookout for knowing glances between her and the priest, but didn't see any.

Father James took me into the rectory and pointed to the bathroom. He said I could let myself out when I was done. I walked carefully behind him, so he wouldn't notice if I staggered a little. I thought it was so cool to be in a rectory by myself that I probably spent a little longer in there than I realized. When I went back to the rehearsal, they had gone through most of the steps without me.

The next morning, I woke up with one of the worst hangovers I ever had.

I couldn't believe it! I had a hangover on Elizabeth's wedding day when I had to be taking pictures, doing all kinds of things at the wedding. I took aspirin, but it didn't help.

My stomach felt so queasy that I didn't even have a cigarette all day, which was highly unusual for me. I didn't dare smoke. I was afraid I would get sick and I was just holding it together as it was.

Miraculously, even though I hadn't really seen much of the rehearsal, I did okay at the wedding. Afterward, when we all lined up on the steps of the church for the picture of the wedding party, I felt like absolute death. With a pounding headache, I curled my lips up in the imitation of a smile and hoped for the best.

To my amazement, just about everyone who sees that picture of the wedding party says I was the prettiest girl in it. You can definitely fool some of the people, some of the time.

But not all the people, all of the time.

* * *

After Elizabeth and Robert had settled into domestic, wedded bliss, I went over to their house one night for drinks. It had been ages since we'd spent any quality time together that Elizabeth and I were looking forward to catching up during cocktail hour.

When I arrived with a six-pack of lite beer, Elizabeth pointed me toward the refrigerator. I appreciated the chance to see what other alcohol might be available, if my beer ran out. They had several bottles of wine. I felt at ease knowing that.

After about an hour, Robert left the room, so Elizabeth and I could talk. I was having a great time. I drank all of my beer in about two hours. I was feeling good. I was talkative and I wasn't slurring my words. It was a good place to be, but still I wanted more alcohol.

When I got up to throw my last beer bottle away, I asked Elizabeth, "Would you mind if I had a glass of wine?"

"You're done with the whole six-pack, Linda? You drank all of those beers in two hours?"

"They were lite beers. They don't get me very buzzed."

Elizabeth took on the tone of some sort of stern parent. "No, Linda. You don't need any more alcohol. How about a glass of water?"

I could feel the anger rise in me. Who did she think she was to monitor me? It was outrageous. I really didn't want to battle with Elizabeth, but I wanted another drink.

Despite what she'd said, I made my way to the kitchen and said, with a bit of an attitude, "It's no problem. I'll get it."

Elizabeth followed me, looking disappointed. "You can have ONE glass of wine. I really shouldn't let you, because you're driving." She poured me a glass herself.

I drank it fast. After the six pack, that one glass of wine made me very buzzed. I was feeling great though. I was high. "Can I have one more glass?" I smiled. I didn't want to stop.

"No," Elizabeth insisted. "You said one and I shouldn't have given you that one glass. You're getting drunk now. I can see that. You're too drunk to drive."

I knew she'd made up her mind. So had I. I wanted more. Elizabeth wasn't going to give it to me, so I went to grab my keys.

Elizabeth was one step ahead of me. She snatched the keys out from under me. They were in her hands.

My face changed. "GIVE ME MY DAMN KEYS," I yelled, raising my voice so she'd give them back to me.

"No."

I lunged at Elizabeth to scare her and throw her off,

then grabbed the keys out of her hands.

I gave her a triumphant look. I had my keys. And I started for the door.

"If you won't give me any wine, I'll go drive myself to get some wine," I yelled, walking defiantly out the front door.

Worried about my safety, Elizabeth followed me out to my car, yelling at me not to get in the car. She knew I was determined to keep drinking. And she was determined not to let me drive when I was drunk.

"Come back inside," she said. "If you give me your keys, I'll give you as much wine as you want."

That was all I wanted to hear.

I gave Elizabeth my keys and went peaceably back inside. There were still a few bottles in the refrigerator. And Elizabeth kept her word. She let me have as much wine as I wanted. I got totally drunk and spent the night in the guest bedroom.

The next morning Elizabeth made me coffee and gave me some aspirin for my nasty headache. She told me she had never seen me like that before and said I shouldn't drink if I acted like that. The secret was out. I'd managed to cover it up at the wedding, but now there was no mistake. Elizabeth knew I had a serious problem with alcohol. She said she would never drink with me again. But I didn't care.

9

Loss

Even during my heaviest drinking years, God was always in the back of my mind. My dad was one of the reasons for that. Every time I talked with him, he mentioned God.

After his accident in Michigan, my father had remained dedicated to God. Whenever Julie and I went up to his house in Cambria for dinner, he'd talk to us about God. He'd tell us that life without an experience of God has no meaning. "If you don't have God," he'd say, "all you have is yourself. Your life is empty."

I truly believed in what he was saying. It's just that I also wanted to drink. I actually looked forward to living a beautiful life with God, later — much later — when alcohol wasn't such a big part of my life. I told myself: "That will be the life I aspire to one day when I don't drink." I would get around to it, but in the meantime, I was busy. Drinking.

But the thought of God was always there. Sometimes, if I found myself alone for a few minutes, I'd take the time to pray. My approach was to be straight with God. I never saw the point in using flowery church prayers or making a big ceremony out of it. I was honest and direct. I'd been told that God appreciated honesty, so that's what He got from me, like it or not.

I talked to God about how I wanted to feel Him more in my life. I said I knew He was there, but I really didn't have much of a feeling for Him. So I asked Him to help me feel Him more. I'd feel so wonderful and encouraged after a good prayer session.

I wanted that feeling to stay with me. And the best way I knew to hang onto a good feeling was to have a couple a beers. So, after a good prayer session, I'd typically head out to the liquor store to buy a six-pack — because I felt so close to God.

The idea was that the beer would help me savor the experience of actually feeling the presence of God. So it always surprised me when, after a few beers, the feeling completely went away. I could never seem to get the balance right.

The truth was, I wanted God *and* alcohol. Both were important to me. When I found I couldn't combine the two, I'd get irritated because it wasn't working out as I'd planned. One rush would follow the other — I'd feel filled with God, then buzzed and drunk, then finally, hung over.

I told myself that maybe it wouldn't happen like that the next time, but it always did. Eventually, I was having two or three hangovers a week. That's when I knew something had to give. Things couldn't continue like this. So I gave up God for awhile until I knew how my drinking would turn out.

* * *

I did listen to a call-in, radio talk show, even while I was drinking hard. The speaker was a spiritual man who talked about topics that were so important to me — how to find peace and tranquility in your life and how to live your spiritual values. Some of my favorite talks were on the importance of meditation and making a connection with God. It was inspiring and made me feel good about life.

The only problem was that it came on Sunday mornings very early — from five o'clock to nine. Bad timing because Saturday night was a heavy drinking night for me. After crashing into bed in a drunken stupor at 3:00 A.M., I was hardly going to get up to listen to a radio show at five, no matter how inspiring it was. You don't need inspiration if you're sound asleep!

But I always regretted missing it. Sometimes I'd be out at a bar on a Saturday night, having a great time, and I'd actually stop for a moment and think, You know, I could stop drinking and go home now.... If I keep drinking, I won't be able to get up in time for my radio show in the morning.

I'd finish my beer and take another drag off my cigarette while I considered it. All around me, I could see people laughing and having a good time. No one in the room was going home anytime soon. So I could walk out now and go to bed early or have another beer and sweeten my buzz. The choice was obvious. After I'd had several drinks, there was no way I could stop anyway. But I still played this little game with myself, week after week.

Instead of picking up my purse to pay my tab, I'd smile at the bartender and point at my empty glass. And she'd start pouring me another one. Then I'd tell myself, Next week I'll get a six-pack and stay home on Saturday night, watching TV. I'll stop after three or four beers and get to bed around ten.

There were so many things wrong with that plan. For one thing, staying home on Saturday night sounded like the most boring, get-a-life idea I'd ever heard. Stopping after three or four beers sounded even worse. It was an empty promise. It was never going to happen. Yet I fell for it every time. Or at least I pretended I did.

I never said to myself, If the radio show comes on Sunday morning before dawn, forget it. It seemed like saying no to the radio show was a way of saying no to God. And I didn't want to do that. So I just kept making promises I didn't keep.

* * *

I always figured God could do something about my drinking, if He wanted to. I never prayed about stopping drinking because truthfully I liked it and didn't want to give it up. I'd be too bored without drinking. Until I found something else to do to fill up my days, I was going to drink.

But I secretly thought that one day God might send me a message to let me know that I had to give it up. I don't know exactly what I was expecting. Not a burning bush or a blinding light with a voice from the heavens. Preachers were always talking about Moses and the Apostle Paul, but you didn't get too many burning bushes or blinding lights these days.

The modern stories of signs from God were more likely to be medical. A doctor tells a man his liver is shot and he's got to give up drinking, so he prays to God for salvation. My liver was fine, as far as I knew, so I didn't know what God might do to get my attention, but I was open to some sort of miracle that would turn my life around and cause me to cut back on my drinking. And the operative phrase of course was "cut back." I never, ever thought of giving up alcohol for good. For me, even cutting back would take a miracle!

It never crossed my mind to feel guilty. Why should I? God had created me and He knew my mind. So He understood that it was crazy to expect me to give up drinking.

As I imagined Him, God was not critical and judgmental — about my drinking or anything else in my life. I'd always seen God as loving and understanding. I believed He was looking out for my good, wanting the best for me and sending me more blessings than I realized every single day. At least that's what I thought before David died.

David was my baby brother. I'd loved him from the moment my parents brought him home from the hospital in a blanket. He was kind and gentle and very, very young. It was inexcusable for God to take him away.

* * *

I'll never forget the day David laughed for the first time. He was a little over twelve months old. I was sitting on the living room floor, playing with him, when he suddenly started laughing. We'd never heard him do that before. And it wasn't just a laugh — it was a belly laugh. The entire family started laughing with him. It was one of the happiest moments I remember.

As he grew up, we became close. I loved watching him grow into a guy who cared about others and was well-liked by his classmates and friends. Even as a young boy, he had a quiet maturity that made it easy for me to talk to him as an adult or friend. And he always liked the fact that I didn't treat him like a kid, but as my equal.

When he was about thirteen, I asked him, "What do you think happens to you when you die?" For a few minutes he was fascinated with the question, trying to come up with an answer, but he couldn't. Then I told him, "It will always be a mystery, won't it? How do we know what happens? We haven't been through it. But we're all going to die some day."

"It's just weird, isn't it?" he said.

* * *

When I got the news David had been killed in a car accident, it was the worst pain I had ever gone through. I knew my life would be changed forever from that day forward. I had seen him the day before. He had gotten his learner's permit for driving. Mom let him drive by the motel to see me. He was excited. He had wanted to drive for a long time and now he was finally getting to. It was his moment of liberation.

"Hey, Linda, I'm driving!" he said, as he came through the door into the office at the Ming Tree Motel. "I got my permit." Our mom came in behind him, beaming proudly at her son.

"Congratulations!" I grinned. We all went outside to see David behind the steering wheel on his first official day as a driver.

"That's a pretty dress you're wearing," he said, as we walked out to the car.

"Oh, I look so fat in this dress!" I exclaimed, looking down at the red stripes that I thought made me look like a circus tent.

David gave me a big hug. "Linda, don't put yourself down. You look great."

When he got into the car, he rested his arm on the open window and turned back to me, smiling, as if to say, "Check me out! Here I am behind the wheel!" I was so proud of him. I went out to the street and watched Mom and David drive off until I couldn't see them anymore. That was the last time I saw David.

I got the call from Julie the morning after David died. She was calling from the Ming Tree and told me David had been in a car accident — a friend was driving his own car too fast. David was a passenger. I went into shock. I had just seen David hours earlier.

Dad and Tish had driven to Santa Barbara the night before from Cambria when they heard about David's accident. They got the call from Mom's new husband Mel and rushed down to Santa Barbara.

I knew it would be difficult for me, but I had to go down to the Ming Tree where everyone was gathered in the motel room where Craig lived. I cried as I drove the few miles to the motel, not caring if anyone saw me. My little brother was dead and I'd never see him again! It couldn't sink in yet. It was too final.

I pulled into the motel parking lot. Julie was standing by the front door to the office. Craig walked out of the motel apartment. He reached out and hugged me with one arm, and embraced Julie with the other. We all stood in the parking lot hugging and crying.

We spent some time with Dad and Tish, and then Craig volunteered to drive us up to Mom's house. We pulled up in front, parked and walked up to the front door and let ourselves in. Mel was sitting in an easy chair in the living room, reading a newspaper. It was apparent he'd been crying.

"Your mother is in the bedroom. I'll get her," said Mel. He came out a few minutes later, with fresh tears in his eyes. "Your mother will be out in a few minutes," he said, then quickly ran downstairs to give us time alone. The old family dog, Puppy, came running up the stairs when she heard us. I pet her and looked into her eyes. She knew something was very wrong.

Julie, Craig and I sat in the living room waiting for Mom to come out. I knew this was going to be one of the hardest visits we'd ever spend together. I needed a drink badly, more than I ever had.

Mom finally opened the door after about a half hour. She was in her bathrobe, holding several Kleenex. "I can't stop crying," she said, and then began to sob uncontrollably. She walked up to the three of us, hugged us and we all cried together.

For the next two years, any memory of David would make me cry. I missed him tremendously. Sometimes the pain was so intense, so hard to bear, that I just kept thinking it would be easier to die.

I started drinking hard the same day, but I couldn't get drunk. For the next several days after his death, I must've had fifteen to twenty beers a day, but I barely even got buzzed. I was in shock and the alcohol didn't have the desired effect. It was a shame, too, because I'd never needed to be drunk like I needed it then.

For years after that, I drank harder and harder to get high. A few times, I drank an entire case of beer (twenty-four beers) in a day. And if you're considering it, let me warn you: A case of beer in a day will give you a very nasty hangover.

Just before losing David, I'd felt closer to God than I had in years, but immediately afterward I stopped talking to God altogether. I was angry at Him for letting David die. He was only sixteen. He had his whole life in front of him. If God had any power at all, He could have prevented that. In my mind, there was no reason for God to let that happen.

* * *

As devastated as he was over David's death, my dad never did blame God in the same way. When they'd learned that David had gotten in a car accident and was in the hospital, my dad and his wife, Letitia, had driven down to Santa Barbara. They stayed in the Ming Tree where I was working.

A day or so later, I went by the motel to be with Dad, but he wasn't there.

"He went walking on the beach to draw close to God," Letitia said.

I was shocked. How could he have anything to do with God after David had been killed? It was just too ridiculous.

A few moments later, when Dad came back to the room, I could see that he had been crying. "Why would you want to be close with God now?" I demanded. "Personally, I've got nothing to say to God now."

"Honey, I think you're wrong," my dad said. "We really need God right now. I understand how you feel about the loss of your brother... I lost my son." With that, he broke down and started crying. The loss was too much for all of us to bear. My dad went into the bathroom for awhile, to be alone and cry. When he came back a few minutes later, he had composed himself and gotten his thoughts together.

"Linda," he said, "I would urge both you and Julie to be open to God right now. Letitia and I will be working for you two throughout these days, sending God's energy to you. That will help, but you've got to reach out to God on your own as well."

I appreciated his intentions, but there was no way that I was going to do that. I knew God could have saved the life of my baby brother and He didn't. Nothing my father said about it could sway me.

Looking back on it now, I wish I'd listened to him. I could have probably saved myself a lot of pain.

* * *

For the next two years, I drank as much as I could stomach and gave God the silent treatment.

When I did decide to start speaking to Him again, I didn't do it right away. I wanted a little bit of lead time. I just opened my mind to the possibility of beginning to talk to God again, whenever it felt right. Even making the decision to break the ice with God made me feel a bit of peace, because I hadn't spoken to God at all for a long time, except to yell at Him when I was drunk.

Then one day, I was home alone and thought I might as well just do it and get it over with. I hadn't started drinking yet that day, so my thoughts were pretty clear. I figured it was as good a time as any.

I sat down on my bed and said, nonchalantly, "God, I haven't talked to you in two years because I've been so pissed off at you for letting David die. I'm still mad at you. I've just decided to stay open. But you're going to have to make the first move. You owe me that. And let me tell you, I need a miracle here, because some days… God… I don't even want to live…"

The drinking had helped dull some of the pain. I knew it and so did God. But it hadn't made me happy for long. Underneath the high was always the low that I was drinking so hard to forget. As I started to think about it, I wanted a drink. "That's it for today, God. Maybe next time we talk I'll be in a better mood."

10

Getting Fired

AFTER DAVID'S DEATH IN 1983, I HAD A NEW REASON TO drink: I needed to drown the pain. And for awhile it looked as if my life was going to make drinking easy. The jobs Julie and I had at the Ming Tree Motel were similar to paid happy hours. We couldn't have drunk more freely on the job if we'd been hired as beer tasters at a brewery.

I was comfortable at the motel. It was almost like a family business. Michael, the manager, had hired my brother Craig and his friend Gary as night managers. They lived in the apartment behind the front office. Julie and I worked as desk clerks, trading off on afternoon and evening shifts.

After Craig and Gary moved out, Michael asked if Julie and I would like to fill their night manager slot. All we had to do to earn our twenty-five dollars a night was to spend the night in the apartment and be on call. We were expected to answer the phone if it rang in the middle of the night, and to be there in case of an emergency.

For a couple of heavy drinkers, it sounded like a dream job. It not only gave us twenty-five dollars to pay for beer and wine, but also it gave us a place to drink it.

If Julie was working the afternoon shift, she'd wait till Michael went home, and then call me. "Happy hour time!" she'd announce. I'd grab my purse and head out the door, stopping off at the liquor store on the way to pick up a six-pack of beer for me and a bottle of wine for Julie. When I worked the afternoon shift, we switched roles. I'd be the one to make the call and she'd pick up the beer. It was the perfect set up. It gave us hours and hours of happy hours.

Unfortunately, we did have nights when there were a lot of interruptions from customers wanting to see the rooms, checking in, losing their keys, needing extra pillows, whatever. Sometimes I felt like saying, "What now? Can't you see I'm drinking?" But usually we got such a kick out of knowing that we could drink and work at the same time, that we considered the customers a minor irritation.

Before long I was spending half the week at the motel, literally being paid to drink. Some nights I drank steadily for the entire shift. If I knew I had to work the office alone, I would make sure not to get drunk. But if I had friends over, I figured one of us would be able to handle the customers, so I let myself drink more.

If a customer complained to Michael that they'd tried to call the office and no one had answered, I'd just tell him I must not have heard the phone because I'd been sleeping too deeply. I'd been unconscious after drinking so many beers was more like it, but that was my little secret. Michael was such a sweetheart and liked our family and was always willing to believe my excuses. I don't think he ever suspected what was going on.

* * *

There was only one night that I really pushed things too far. I didn't know it at the time, but it would be my last night at the motel.

Earlier in the day, I'd invited Bob, a guy I'd been seeing, to stop by the apartment at the motel around eight. I didn't really like Bob all that much. He used to love to sit for hours with the TV remote in his hand, surfing the channels, but never watching a show. It was annoying. I would sit there watching him do this and think, "How can I be with such a loser?" He had no hobbies, no interests outside of his job. I didn't either, of course, but I wasn't critical of myself. I was critical of Bob.

When he told me he'd drop by, I said, "Okay. Bring me a six-pack of beer. And, oh, bring something for yourself too."

By the time Bob got there, Julie and I had been drinking for hours. I'd already had about eight beers. I wasn't drunk, but I was getting there fast. We had the music turned up in the apartment and the TV on. Bob's ice-cold beer made things even better. Julie decided to head home. But Bob was in a lively mood and I felt like a party. It was turning out to be a great night.

And then I heard the bell on the counter in the office.

I'd been having so much fun drinking that I'd forgotten to close up.

The front door was unlocked and there was obviously a customer at the counter waiting for me. I couldn't quite get a fix on the idea. I didn't lock the door? My thoughts seemed to float in slow motion in my head. Nothing was clear. But I knew it was my job to answer that bell. So I got up off the bed. All of a sudden, the room, which had been perfectly normal before, started spinning. I hadn't realized how drunk I was.

Each step I took required my full concentration. All I kept thinking was, "Maintain, maintain..."

When I reached the counter, there was a tall, timid-looking man waiting on the other side. His hand was poised to press the bell again when he saw me.

My lips moved to say, "Can I help you, sir?" but nothing came out. And I decided that didn't bother me.

"How much are your rooms?" the man asked.

Now that I looked at him, he seemed incredibly timid. Almost mousy. I wondered what he was doing out, so late at night, a timid little man like this.

I knew the prices of the rooms. They were forty-six to one hundred dollars. A single was forty-six dollars and a suite was one hundred dollars. I said so too. But the words didn't sound right. Listening to myself, I couldn't even understand what I'd said.

The timid man took a step back, scowled and looked a little alarmed.

I tried it again. "Mnrffrst ... arlllewfant..." Nothing. It had finally happened: I was so drunk I couldn't talk. Every time I tried, a bunch of gibberish came out.

I blinked hard and shook my head. I added gestures for emphasis. Nothing helped.

Finally the timid man's alarm gave way to sad recognition. He knew I was drunk. I could see it on his face. He glanced out wistfully toward the rooms for a moment, then slowly picked up his suitcase and let himself out.

We'd lost a customer. I felt a little bad about that. But mainly, I was mad at myself because I couldn't talk. That had never happened before.

Somehow I made it around the counter and locked the door. By the time the man's car had driven away I was over it.

Back to drinking! No more interruptions!

I staggered back to the apartment, hoping to make out a little with Bob, now that we were officially closed, but Bob had his jacket on. Apparently, the idea of making out with someone who was too drunk to talk didn't appeal to him. He was ready to go. It was just as well, I told myself. All this walking and talking — or trying to talk — was making me queasy. "All right then. Hurry up! GO!" I shouted, suddenly regaining my ability to form basic words. I leaned into him hard, shoving him out the door.

It amazed me that I could be having a good time drinking one minute, and then a second later feel like I was going to puke. Whenever that happened, other people had to go. I needed to take care of myself immediately.

With Bob gone, I went back to the bed and lay down on top of the covers, then I reached over and turned on the fan. As long as I had cool air blowing directly on me, I could stave off getting sick most of the time. Even in winter, when it was cold, I still had to have the fan blowing on me. Hours after I'd fallen asleep, I'd wake up freezing. I'd drag myself out of bed, shivering, put on a couple of winter nightgowns, pile on several blankets and then crawl back in to get warm. But even then I wouldn't turn off the fan.

That night the fan didn't help. I fell asleep as soon as my eyes closed, but when I woke up the next morning, I was just as sick. The clock next to the bed said 10:00 A.M. I couldn't believe it. I never slept that late.

My stomach felt like I'd been drinking sewer water and my head was about to explode, but I had to get up. Michael was working the morning shift. He would already be in the office by now. I couldn't lie around in bed — especially not hung over.

It felt like I was still a little drunk from the night before. I'd always heard that it was possible to be technically drunk the next day after a night of overdrinking. And I'd definitely had too much to drink the night before. As I got up and pulled on a fresh pair of jeans, I told myself I would never drink like that on the job again. And even more importantly I couldn't get so drunk that I forgot to lock the door and let random customers wander in!

I took a quick look in the mirror. My eyes were a little strained, but they weren't bloodshot. And, after all, I had a throbbing headache. So of course I looked a little pale. Ashen, maybe, but who was going to notice?

I brushed my teeth a second time and popped in a breath mint, so Michael wouldn't smell alcohol on me when I left. Then I fluffed up my hair a little more and practiced a cheerful smile in a mirror. It was a little scary, with my eyes looking so bleak, but it would do.

* * *

When I walked into the office, Michael was at the counter looking over the receipts from the previous night. He glanced up at me and looked back down nervously before I could beam him with my cheerful smile.

"Hi, Michael," I said cautiously, trying to figure out whether something was wrong.

"Linda…" he said, turning his back to me to put the receipts in the drawer. "Was it busy last night?" His voice kind of trembled as he said it.

"Not too bad."

Something was wrong. Had that timid man called the main office and reported me? Was there something wrong with the receipts? Michael was definitely not himself.

I hesitated briefly, wondering if I should hang around and figure out what was bothering him. But my stomach growled and I started thinking about the breakfast special at Sambo's. Those hash browns were so good. What I really needed was some food and coffee to get rid of that nasty churning feeling in my stomach.

"Okay, well, I'll see you later, Michael," I said, walking toward the door.

And then he blurted it out: "I'm sorry to have to be the one to tell you, Linda. But you and Julie are being let go."

Even as dense and out of it as I felt at that moment, I knew this was not good.

I said the only thing I could think of. "What?"

"I know. Look, I hate having to tell you this. It was Dennis's decision."

Dennis was the owner of the motel, but we hardly ever saw him. Michael ran the place and half his employees were members of my family! What he said was finally starting to get through to me. I'd been working at the Ming Tree, off and on, since I was sixteen. And now, twelve years later, I wake up one morning, with a blazing headache, and it's over? Just like that? The same day? This sucked!

"I'll need your master key," Michael said, all business now.

Half-dazed, I reached into my pocket and pulled out the keys. My hands had been shaking when I walked into the room, but now they were shaking so hard I couldn't get the master key off the key chain. Finally I handed the keys to Michael. "Will you take it off? I can't do it."

Michael was the one who looked pale now. He may not have handled it in the most sensitive way, but I knew this was difficult for him. He took the key chain out of my trembling hand and removed the master key.

"Here's the thing," he said, the kindness returning to his voice. "Dennis's sons are moving up here next week to learn the motel business from their dad. He wants them to take the apartment and live on the premises. So what could I do? Dennis said I needed to either let you or Julie go. I thought it would be too difficult to pick one of you, so I said we should let you both go."

He handed me back my key chain. It felt a lot lighter. We stood there looking at each other for a minute. There was nothing else to say.

* * *

I was afraid of what was going to happen next. It wasn't because of the money. I still had quite a bit of money saved up and I knew I could collect unemployment for weeks. But I was deeply afraid of being bored most of the day. What would I do with all that free time?

I had no hobbies, no passions and no goals. One of the things I dreaded most was waking up in the morning and having a whole day in front of me with nothing to do. I couldn't stand to be alone. So I always tried to be doing something with other people — like my boyfriend at the time or strangers in a bar if need be — to keep myself occupied.

The two days I'd had off from the motel every week had been almost unbearable. I'd get so bored not being at work, that I'd try to find a way to stop by and spend time at the motel for awhile. As soon as I got there, I'd be surrounded by people I knew. After twelve years, a lot of the guests that came to the motel would ask for me personally. We chatted like old friends. The motel had been the focus of my work and social life since high school. In the rest of my life, I didn't know what to do with myself. I couldn't wait until I had to go back to work.

The only way I'd ever found to cope with my days off was to drink more heavily the night before. That way, I could spend most of the next day sleeping it off or lying around the house, nursing a hangover. I'd wake up, have coffee, shower, do a few errands and then the loneliness would set in. That's when I'd ask Julie, whom I was living with at the time, if she'd like to make plans to have cocktail hour with me. Her answer was almost always yes and I felt secure knowing I had just found a way to kill several hours that day. I wouldn't be bored or lonely after all. No matter what, I knew I could always kill a couple of hours drinking.

The truth was, work had kept me from noticing my life was going nowhere. I had no interests. I wasn't reaching any goals. I wasn't thinking of my future at all. Most of the guys I dated were almost interchangeable. And if I was with friends, we were usually too drunk to make a real connection.

With a job, I'd managed to stay occupied enough to keep from feeling the emptiness of my life. Now that emptiness was all I could feel.

* * *

After I left Michael in the office, I picked up a sandwich and beer and went to find Julie to tell her the news. She was at the city college taking a class to learn sign language. When I peered in the doorway, I could see Julie on the far side of a room filled with students, all signing to each other. It really did look fun. Maybe I would learn sign language … someday.

I looked at the clock. There were only about ten minutes left in the class. So I went outside to smoke a cigarette and waited. When class was over, Julie came out with the other students and I caught her eye. She looked concerned. "Why are you here?"

"We got fired," I said, getting right to the point. Then we went outside and sat on a bench on the school grounds and I told her the whole story. We both agreed we'd miss our cushy jobs a lot.

When we went back to collect our stuff from the motel, I picked up a radio, a toothbrush and a few clothes. Julie dragged out seven empty wine bottles she'd hidden in the back of the kitchen cupboards. She came walking out into the living room, trying to hold onto all of them at once.

"You kept those bottles in the cupboards? Are you serious?" I said. "That was an amazingly stupid idea! What if Dennis looked in those cupboards? It's his place. He has every right to do it."

"Well, I couldn't throw them away at the office. He'd definitely find out then," she said, throwing the bottles into the trunk of her car.

For awhile, we wondered whether Dennis had found the bottles or not. But no one ever let on that they knew we'd been drinking. And Dennis's sons really did take over the family business after we left. So we figured Michael was telling us the truth.

To commemorate our final moments, we'd decided to drink while we picked up our stuff. After all this time, Michael had never seen either of us holding a drink. When he came in and saw me with a beer in my hand, it felt like a little secret confession to me. It was actually very liberating. The truth was out. Whether he knew it or not.

We said goodbye to everyone and Michael gave us our

last checks with two weeks' paid vacation for each of us. Then we went home. Another chapter in our lives had closed.

*   *   *

Before long, I filled up some of the empty hours with temp jobs. For several years, I'd been signed up with many of the temporary employment agencies in town. I'd take a job for a day or two, during slow periods at the motel. The agencies had always been eager to place me because I interviewed well and kept their customers happy.

I knew that if I were going to take a lot of agency assignments, I'd have to coordinate my drinking more carefully. It was just too difficult to work when I was hung over. My mind was dull. New tasks were harder to grasp and remember. I wasn't at my best. So whenever I planned to work within the next few days, I'd tried to not drink at all.

As soon as I left the motel, I let the agencies know that I would be available for longer assignments. Within a few weeks, Ellen, a placement person from one of the best agencies in town called to offer me a job at a local hospital.

"It's forty hours a week for three months," she said. "I know that's more hours than we talked about. Would you be interested?"

It was a good job. I knew that. But I just couldn't make myself agree to forty hours a week for three months. It felt like signing up for a chain gang. I looked for a reason to say no. When she told me what it paid, I said I might be interested, but I'd have to have more money than they were offering.

Within an hour Ellen called me back. "I told them I recommended you very highly and you were worth the extra money. They've agreed to pay another fifty cents an hour. You've got the job."

"Great," I said, feeling the enthusiasm drain out of me.

I should have been ecstatic, but I wasn't. I couldn't help thinking how much I'd miss my beers.

The whiny voice in my head started in. Why did I take this job? I certainly didn't want it. I wondered what she'd do if I called and cancelled. How could I possibly go without drinking during the week for three months?

But this was nonsense. I had to snap out of this. I'd accepted the job. Now I had to take it. It was just forty hours a week. Other people did it all the time. I could do it. Besides, the paycheck would be nice.

Gradually I calmed myself down. I started to see that it just might work out. Maybe I'd even like it. Starting the next day I was going to be a full-time worker for three months. What was wrong with that? Things would be fine. No, better than fine. I was happy.

To prove it, I invited Julie to come downtown with me to one of our favorite bars to celebrate. It had the best happy hour in town. "Now, I have to go home by five at the latest and I'm just having a couple of drinks," I told her. "I start my new job in the morning, so I have to be fresh. Promise me you'll remind me when it's time to go and I'll buy you a drink."

Julie promised, but when we arrived at the bar, the place was hopping with excitement. I ran into some party friends I hadn't seen in awhile and I started drinking fast. Five o'clock came and went. When Julie reminded me that it was time to go, I told her she could go home if she wanted. I'd be along later. I figured I could go to work the first day with a slight hangover. I'd done it before.

Besides, it was going to be a long time before I could party like this again. Soon I'd be getting up early every morning and going into work at a real job. Unless I wanted to end up sneaking sips from a flask in the corridors like some hopeless alcoholic when the nurses weren't looking, I'd have to swear off drinking during the week and hold out for weekends. Basically I told myself I wouldn't be able to drink from Sunday until Friday night — six long days every week for twelve weeks. The very idea set off a kind of quiet panic in me.

I stayed at the bar drinking nonstop for seven hours. Then my friends and I went to a dance club around the corner. We laughed and danced and had the time of our lives till the doors closed at 1:00 A.M.

When I got home, I set my alarm for six thirty. Only about five hours' sleep, but I'd sleep hard with all this alcohol in me. And then I'd have plenty of time to have coffee, take a shower and get to the hospital by eight thirty Friday morning for my first day of work.

When the alarm went off the next morning, I felt like I'd only been asleep for about an hour. My eyes were puffy and swollen. When I opened them, the light sent stabs of pain through my head. I felt like I had a migraine. When I sat up, a wave of nausea swept over me and knocked me back down again. I had to face the fact that I wouldn't be going to work that day. What a drag. A three-month job and I'd have to call in sick the first day.

I knew that wouldn't go over well with Ellen, but — hey — people get sick all the time, don't they?

When the agency opened at 8:00 A.M. I was afraid to make the call, but I didn't have any choice. "Ellen, this is Linda Joy Allan calling. I woke up with a terrible flu. I'm so sorry, but I won't be able to go that hospital job today. Can you ask them if I can come in Monday? I'm sure I'll be better by then and I really, really want this job."

There was silence for a few moments. When Ellen spoke, her voice was stony. "I'll call you back after I talk to the hospital. But they specifically told me they needed someone to start today."

Well, that was settled. I'd known she wouldn't be happy. I was letting her down. It happens. But I was sure they'd wait until Monday. It was a hospital, for god's sake. They deal with sick people all the time.

Assuming everything was fine, I fell back asleep for twenty minutes, till the phone woke me up. It was Ellen. "The hospital needs someone to start today. We're sending another one of our people," she said. "I have to tell you, Linda, I'm very disappointed."

That agency never did call me again. But I didn't even care. There were other agencies in town. And if I were more careful and took shorter-term jobs, getting work would never be a problem. I hung up the phone and went back to sleep.

11

Drinking Down the Pain

ONCE MY HEAVY DRINKING KICKED IN, THE PEOPLE WHO loved me tried to intervene. At first, they'd quietly suggest that "maybe I'd had enough for the night." Soon afterward, they began to suspect that I had a serious drinking problem. They'd tell me how worried they were about how much I was drinking. They seemed to think that if they pointed it out to me, I might cut back. What they didn't realize was, I was just getting started…

One night, when Julie and I were out of town in Yorba Linda, I drank so much that I literally didn't care what happened to me. I could have easily put my life in danger. In the weeks and years to come I would do that often. It still amazes me that I survived those years in one piece.

* * *

After the Ming Tree Motel, I drifted from one temporary job to another. My mother's husband was a college counselor. He said there was a place in Yorba Linda that had a great two-day intensive test that helped identify which careers would best match your skills and interests. "It won't just tell you what you should do," he told me. "It'll tell you which careers you might really enjoy."

Since I still had no outside interests, other than drinking, I joked with Julie that the test would probably show I'd be an excellent bartender or cocktail waitress. But I had nothing better to do, so I was willing to give it a try —

especially when my mom said she'd pay the $125 for the test and for the two nights in a hotel. If nothing else, it would be a couple of free days out of town. But I didn't want to go alone, so Julie came along for the ride.

Yorba Linda is a small town, only twenty square miles wide, about three hours south of Santa Barbara. Its sole claim to fame is the Richard M. Nixon Library. Other than that, it's just one more quiet little community next to Anaheim, that sprawling flatland of industrial buildings and freeway overpasses.

All the hotels in a chain look so much alike, that once we checked into the hotel, it almost didn't matter where we were. I glanced around to find the bar while we were still at the front desk, and found it exactly where I thought it would be.

"Why don't we have a few drinks before dinner?" I asked Julie, nodding toward the bar.

Julie smiled. "It'd be a shame to miss happy hour," she agreed.

With the test the next morning, I knew I shouldn't drink more than two beers — three at the most. I wanted to be alert and at my best the next day. This was about finding a job that would make me happy. If the test could point me in the right direction, I might be able to really make something wonderful of my life. Even though I'd have to wait a few weeks for the results, I was starting to get excited about the prospect of taking the test.

So I made myself another promise: I will limit myself to a few beers. Then we'll have dinner and I'll go right to bed. I'll set the alarm early enough to have time for coffee in the morning, so I will be refreshed and ready for the test. There was only one thing I hadn't considered. After a few beers, I wasn't going to care about the plan anymore.

Julie and I sat at the bar and had a few drinks. Because it was happy hour, they served us free hors d'oeuvres. Silly as they are, I was especially fond of those "pigs in a blanket."

They were like mini hot dogs, so small you could almost plop two of them in your mouth at a time. And they were very filling. Once I'd eaten those for awhile, I wasn't hungry any longer. So much the better! "I don't feel like eating dinner now, do you?" I asked Julie. "The Holiday Inn is just across the street. Why don't we go over for their happy hour instead?" I was feeling in a party mood.

I always knew I had to eat at some point when I was drinking, or I'd have a hangover the next day for sure. But I was careful not to eat so much that I was full. If I was full, I didn't enjoy drinking much, and my buzz would wear off.

The Holiday Inn had a happy hour special of two for one drinks. Things were looking up. Every time I guzzled two glasses of beer, I only paid one low, happy hour price. And I loved it. Welcome to Yorba Linda!

Julie was getting the same deal, but she was drinking about half as fast. After an hour or so, she said, bluntly, "You know, your test is tomorrow morning. If you keep drinking like this, you're going to be hung over. We should go back to our hotel."

I didn't mind going back to our hotel. I could eat a few more of those pigs in a blanket. They didn't have them at the Holiday Inn. When we got to the hotel, Julie headed up to the room. "I'm just going to grab a few more hors d'oeuvres," I told her. "I'll be up in a little while."

Julie gave me a look but didn't say anything. She spent more time with me than the rest of my family, so she learned sooner than anybody else that it was pointless to try to get in my way when I really wanted to drink. She took the room key, but promised to be there to let me in when I came up.

It couldn't have been more perfect. I loved going to bars out of town because they were filled with people who didn't know me. It gave me such freedom. Somehow, I felt bolder when I was alone. I could easily strike up conversations with strangers. It was a lot more fun.

* * *

When I walked back into the bar, I took a stool and waved to the bartender. "Back again!" I smiled. "Another Miller Lite, please." I snatched a little pig in a blanket from the tray and looked around the room to see who was there.

A man who was much older than I struck up a conversation with me. He wasn't my type at all, but he bought me several drinks while I was there. Before long, the band arrived and live music started to play. "Let's dance," the man said.

I knew that if the band had arrived, it was getting later than I thought. "I'd better go get the room key from my sister," I told him.

"You can do that in a minute," he said. "First, a dance…"

By that time, my head was spinning with alcohol. It made me compliant. We had a couple of dances and a few more drinks after that before I remembered the key again. Then I promised I'd be right back and pulled myself away.

It was a miracle I remembered our room number. I took the elevator up, then staggered up to our door and knocked. It was a minute or so before Julie answered. I'd woken her up. I'd been having such a good time with my new friend that I had no idea what time it was.

"Where is the key?" I said, leaning against the doorsill to the room.

Julie squinted at me for a moment, trying to wake up. "No. No key. You're drunk. You need to get some sleep. Your test is tomorrow. That's why we're here. Now, come on in and go to bed."

"Look, I told my friend I'd be right back. He's waiting for me. Just give me the key!" Julie was really starting to get on my nerves.

"No, I won't give you the key. You'll just lose it."

That did it. Now she was insulting me. I hated when anyone gave me their "holier-than-thou" attitude. I pushed past Julie and started picking things up in the room, looking for the key.

"Where is the key?" I demanded, tossing stuff around. The more I searched the angrier I got. I started throwing everything on the floor or across the room. I was livid. But I couldn't find the key. Where had she hidden it?

"If you don't give me the key, I'm not coming home tonight," I swore. I was always so dramatic when I was drunk and angry. Threatening was my favorite tactic. Even if I didn't mean what I was saying, it always felt so righteous to say it.

"I'm not giving it to you, Linda," Julie insisted. "And if you leave now, I won't open the door when you get back. I mean it."

She was threatening me now? It was too much. "Fine!" I said and walked out the door.

* * *

As the elevator took me back down to the bar, I smiled. Knowing Julie, she wouldn't be able to go back to sleep now because she'd be nervous about what might happen to me. Served her right for threatening me. I happily made my way back to the bar and found my "friend" waiting. He bought me yet another drink, then took my hand and led me to the dance floor. One of my favorite love songs by Lionel Ritchie had started to play. I closed my eyes.

The man in the bar pulled me closer, dancing slowly and rubbing against me. Lost in my memories, I momentarily forgot who I was dancing with. When he started kissing me, it didn't surprise me at all. I loved kissing Chris. He had such beautiful, blond hair — a surfer's blond, bleached by the sun and the salt in the waves. I reached up to run my hand through it, as he held me tight, but this guy was nearly bald!

I opened my eyes and looked at him. It wasn't Chris. It was some older man I didn't know. That guy who'd been buying me drinks all night. I snapped out of my affectionate mood. The alcohol hit me and I started feeling like I was going to be sick.

Without another word, I pulled away from him, picked up my purse and walked right out the hotel door. There was really nowhere else to go, but the fresh air made me feel a little better. I sat down on the steps and lit up a cigarette.

The man in the bar followed me outside.

"Leave me alone," I snapped at him, still disgusted that he wasn't Chris.

"Hey, don't talk to me like that," he said. "I bought you drinks and you seemed to be having a good time."

"I'm sick. Just go away," I said, curtly, taking a drag off my cigarette. At least the man had the good sense to leave.

* * *

As the hotel door swung shut behind him, I started to cry. I hated my life. Nothing was working out right. Here I was, drunk in an unfamiliar city, I'd had a fight with my sister, I didn't know what to do with my life and I missed David tremendously.

It was late at night so there was no one outside the hotel. I sat there, whimpering, in peace for awhile. But the cigarette was making me sick.

I stood up and threw the rest of my cigarette on the ground, then I started walking. I didn't know where I was going. I just started walking.

Small towns like Yorba Linda are family towns. Most of the residents tuck their kids into bed at a decent hour and then go to sleep themselves. There's not a lot of night life. If you do encounter someone lurking around a quiet street at night, the chances are they are up to no good.

Ignoring that fact, I headed off the hotel property down

a dark street. I knew I could be mugged or attacked, alone in a strange city in the middle of the night, but it didn't bother me. I was completely wrapped up in my own thoughts and started to cry again. I just didn't care about anything. If something "bad" happened to me, so be it. At least it would end the pain. Maybe I was even secretly hoping something would happen to me and I'd die. If David could die, I told myself, I didn't mind dying too.

From the moment I'd left the hotel, a guy I didn't know had been following me. I'd vaguely heard his footsteps, but they hadn't really registered. I was too busy thinking about David and how much I missed him. But when I'd walked for a block or so and was out of sight of the hotel, the guy picked up his pace and started toward me. I could hear him coming, but I felt like I was fast asleep and someone was calling out to me in a dream, trying to wake me.

"Excuse me!" he shouted, as he grabbed hold of my arm. "Excuse me, Miss!"

When I turned to look at him, my eyes were bleary and it was dark, but he looked like he was about my own age. "Listen," he said, kindly, "I don't think you should be wandering around out here by yourself. Why don't we go back to the hotel for awhile?"

He was cute and friendly, so I quickly agreed. He still had a hold on my arm and when he started leading me back to the hotel, I politely followed along. We sat on the steps so I could smoke another nauseating cigarette. He listened to me cry for a few minutes about how unhappy I was in my life. I told him I missed my brother so much and I just didn't care about anything anymore and that I just wanted to die.

This stranger listened to me like an old friend. I don't know who he was. All I know is, when I needed someone to listen to me babble on and on, he was there for me. Then he walked me up to my room and Julie let me in. I never saw him again after that.

It makes me wonder how many times I was protected from an evil fate when I drank myself into oblivion. This guy said he'd been watching me in the bar and had been worried when he saw me wander away from the hotel, so he came after me. But I'd never noticed him in the bar. What kindness it took for him to go out into the darkness to help a stranger and make sure I got back safely to my room. Who knows what kind of danger I might have been in that night, if he hadn't come along. I always thought I was protected somehow… maybe by angels? I'll never know.

* * *

Before too long, word of these kinds of escapades made their way back to my family. I was always trying to keep them a secret, but since I was so unaware of my actions when I was drunk, my efforts were not too successful. Anyone who had been paying the least bit of attention to my life would've realized that it completely revolved around alcohol.

Even when Julie and I drove up to see our dad in Cambria, the first thing we thought of was getting drinks along the way. Cambria was 150 miles away from Santa Barbara. You can drive past a lot of bars in 150 miles. Julie and I thought it would be fun to go have drinks all along the way, in places we'd never been. New bars offered novelty, excitement and new bartenders.

"You know what's weird about a new bar?" I said to Julie. "The bartender actually has to ask, 'What can I get you?'" We both laughed.

Just about two miles outside of Cambria, we stopped at a cute little motel with a restaurant and bar. We knew we could only have two drinks, no matter what, since we didn't want our dad to be able to detect that we'd been drinking. We both opted for wine. We could get more buzzed with two glasses of wine than two glasses of beer.

It was fun to be doing something on the sly. Stopping at a bar was our secret and getting buzzed was our secret. For me, getting away with little secrets made the whole day a lot more enjoyable.

* * *

When Julie and I arrived at our dad's house, Dad helped us take our luggage out to the guesthouse. It was a small house on the back of his property, where Julie and I always stayed when we were there. With one bedroom with two twin beds and a bath, it was the perfect size for us.

As Dad led Julie out the back door, I took a peek in the refrigerator. When I saw that there was quite a lot of unopened wine, I relaxed. I felt more secure knowing that there was some alcohol around. Dad liked to have a drink every so often and, most likely, the extra wine meant that he had planned on having our own little happy hour that night. If he didn't, I decided I would push for it.

After we unpacked our things, Julie and I sat around in the main house, talking with Dad and Letitia, whom we'd all started calling "Tish." The conversation was pleasant enough, but there was really only one thing on my mind. Late in the afternoon I couldn't stand the suspense any longer, so I asked him point blank. "Are we going to have happy hour tonight?"

"Sure," Dad said. "We can have happy hour. Would you like some wine or would you girls like to go to the liquor store and buy something else?"

Julie and I smiled at each other. This was even better than I'd hoped. I was elated. Not only could I go out and buy some beer, but when I ran out of beer, there was plenty of wine as a back-up.

Since Julie only wanted the wine, Tish and I drove to the liquor store together. I got my six-pack and popped open a beer the minute we got home. Dad and Tish started talking

to us about God and philosophical ideas. I became talkative
and it seemed like Dad was pleased that I had taken such an
interest in spiritual things. I was in a fantastic mood.

The only distraction was that, every time I opened a
new beer, Julie and I had to step outside to have a cigarette
because Dad didn't want us smoking in the house. He lived
right on the beach and it got really cold after the sun went
down. But every twenty minutes or so, we'd interrupt our
conversation to get up, put on our coats and go outside in the
cold to smoke.

"What's the definition of ecstasy?" I asked Julie as we
stood outside shivering and smoking our cigarettes with our
drinks in hand.

"Having a drink in one hand and a cigarette in the
other!" she laughed, quoting our own little definition of ecstasy.

"That's right," I said, taking a satisfied drag on my
cigarette.

As soon as I'd finished that cigarette, my sixth beer
was half gone. I hadn't been paying too much attention to how
fast I'd been drinking because normally my main concern was
running out of alcohol. This time I was very aware of the wine
in the fridge. There was no need to slow down because I knew
I could always switch to wine when my beer ran out. And that
time had come.

Six beers usually lasted three hours but this time they
were gone in two. We'd had two glasses of wine on the way and
I hadn't eaten since breakfast, but I told myself that I was only
a little bit drunk — nothing that anybody else would notice.
Typically, as my blood alcohol level rose, so did my level of
confidence. I was having a great time, chatting with Dad and
Tish and hiding how drunk I was. Any time I pretended I
wasn't drunk, I had no way of knowing if I was convincing or
not. But I thought I was clever enough to fool people.

One of my best tactics was to speak slowly, so I
wouldn't slur my words. Even though talking very slowly is a

dead giveaway that someone's drunk, I liked to think that it was my own carefully crafted ruse.

But I soon found that, no matter how slowly I enunciated, there were some words that I simply could not say when I was drunk. For instance, I could never say the word "literally" if I was truly drunk. It was just too complex. My tongue felt thick when I said it. So it always came out "leerally." At first, I'd give it a few earnest tries, but that only made it more obvious that I couldn't say the word.

So I came up with a new tactic: I gave that word up entirely when I was drunk. I wouldn't go anywhere near it. Who needed to say "literally" anyway? That wasn't the only word I had to give up. There were several others too that I had to completely omit from my vocabulary when I was drunk. I convinced myself that if I simply avoided those words and spoke more slowly, no one would be able to tell I was drunk.

* * *

When I went to Dad's refrigerator to start on the wine, I had just reached the point where speaking slowly was able to get me by. After one glass of wine, I was over the edge — really slurring my words, whether I spoke slowly or not. The wine hit me hard and fast.

I drained the glass quickly and was ready for more. Grabbing onto the armrest, I pulled myself up off the sofa and staggered back toward the refrigerator. The room seemed to tilt a little bit under my feet and I wandered off to the right of the door. My dad was there to intercept me, before I made it to the kitchen.

"Linda, you've had enough, don't you think?"

"Aw, Dad, I'm having such a great time. Just a little more…" He was holding onto me. I tried to push past him, but he wasn't having it.

"No, Linda. You're drunk. That's enough. No more wine."

I tried to laugh it off casually, but the laugh that came out sounded a little wild, even to me. "Dad! I'm not drunk!" What a ridiculous idea! I was sure my casual laughter would've made that perfectly clear... if only my laugh had sounded a little less frantic. "I'm buzzed, not drunk! It's not a problem. One more glass of wine and that's all."

I pulled away from him and walked steadily toward the refrigerator. My mind had already moved on to the next step. What was I going to say to get the next glass of wine after this one? Maybe I could tell him I was going to bed, then sneak back into the kitchen while the others were in the living room talking ...

My dad suddenly stepped between me and the refrigerator. Whoa. I wasn't expecting that.

"No," he said firmly. "You'll ruin our good time. I'm going to have to say no."

Tish was over at the stove and glanced at me with an apologetic look, but continued making the dinner. Dad pulled me gently from the refrigerator and led me back toward the living room. On the way, we passed Julie, headed toward the refrigerator. I reeled around in my dad's arms to see what she was doing ... SHE WAS POURING HERSELF ANOTHER GLASS OF WINE.

I was outraged. "What? Julie can have more, but I can't?"

"Julie's not drunk," my dad insisted.

Well, it's all a matter of interpretation, isn't it? I thought.

I just glared at him. Everyone was ganging up on me. I was in no mood for any more friendly discussions in the living room. "I'm going back to my room," I said, sulking.

"Linda, you're welcome to have dinner with us or you can take your dinner to the guest house and eat alone, if you'd like," my dad said. "But I won't allow you to ruin the mood in the house because you didn't get what you wanted."

I didn't even answer him. I stormed out of the house, headed back to the guest house and slammed the door. I was going to stay locked inside for the rest of the night, but I needed a cigarette.

I zipped up my coat and went back outside. Standing outside the guest house, I smoked my cigarette and thought about how cold it was. I was always colder, anyway, when I was drunk and hadn't had anything to eat. Now I was absolutely freezing. It didn't help that I could see the three of them sitting in the warm living room, laughing and talking. What a miserable day.

There wasn't a clock in the room, but I figured it was about seven thirty or eight. I knew Dad wouldn't come knocking on my door later to try to persuade me to go join them for dinner. That wasn't his style. When I was drunk, he would just as soon not have me join them anyway. I lay down on the bed and pulled the covers over me. With the alcohol pumping through my veins, I fell asleep within minutes. So I never ate dinner at all. I didn't even hear Julie when she came in later that night.

* * *

In the morning I woke up with a nasty hangover. God, what was I going to say to Dad and Tish? I'd felt so self-righteous and betrayed the night before. Now, I just felt embarrassed.

Before I could even decide what to say, I needed a cup of coffee. Dad always left the kitchen door unlocked when we stayed over so we could go in and get coffee in the morning. I went in quietly, hoping no one would be up yet. If I could have a few minutes to wake up and get caffeine into my system, I might be able to shake off a little of my hangover before I faced them.

I paused and listened carefully when I stepped inside. There was no sign of life. The coffee machine was ready to go.

My dad had left a note saying, "Just push the button," so I did.

As the coffee was brewing, I tried to think of what to do. It was definitely going to be uncomfortable when I saw my dad. Should I apologize? Should he apologize? What could I say so we could put it behind us and forget about the whole thing?

As soon as the coffee was ready, I took a cup back to my room. Julie was stepping out of the shower. "Linda, you were so drunk last night! Dad and Tish were asking me all these questions about your drinking…" She rolled her eyes.

Great. Now Dad and Tish were worrying about me. I didn't want people worrying about me. It was no one's business if I drank too much. Everybody does that sometimes. "What questions? What did you tell them?"

"Nothing," Julie promised, drying her hair with the towel. "I told them they should to talk to you about it, if they wanted answers."

"You know what?" I said, chugging down the rest of my coffee. "Let's just go. I don't need the whole drinking lecture from him. I have a splitting headache. We can pack our things and be out of here before Dad even gets up. Okay?"

"You know we can't leave without saying something to Dad and Tish," Julie said.

I agreed. We couldn't just take off without saying "thank you" and "goodbye." I needed another cup of coffee anyway before I saw Dad.

As soon as I stepped back into the kitchen, I knew it was over. My dad was up. He was sitting at the table, nursing his own cup of coffee. The tension in the air was uncomfortable. I tried to make a little morning small talk, but he didn't fall for it. He cut me off in the middle of some lame remark about the weather this time of year.

"Before I saw you drunk last night, I knew that you had… a problem with alcohol…" he said. I could see Dad was choosing his words carefully. "But I didn't know how bad it was." When he looked up at me, I was surprised to see he wasn't angry or blaming. I didn't feel like he was punishing me or ganging up on me, as I'd felt he was the night before. His eyes were filled with sadness. "You know, your grandmother — my mother — was an alcoholic. Seven out of nine of her siblings were alcoholics too." My dad looked like he was going to cry.

In 1972, my father's mother committed suicide. She shot herself with Grandpa's gun and left a suicide note, blaming Grandpa for her death. When I was snooping around her basement in the days afterward, I came across several empty bottles of hard liquor, hidden away so Grandpa wouldn't find them.

It didn't surprise me, since I have vivid memories of Grandma and the special errands we used to go on, when I stayed at her house as a little girl. The errands had an air of mystery and urgency about them that made them seem important and exciting. It felt like an emergency — something we had to do. A secret adventure. And there was always the sense that, if someone caught us doing it, there would be hell to pay.

We'd make sure no one was looking, then the two of us would sneak into her car and rush out on "an errand." I'd be in the back seat, holding on for dear life, while she'd be in the front, singing or chatting away, as she drove, weaving and lurching over the lines in the road. Our errands always took us to the liquor store.

Now it was all starting to come together. I knew a tendency toward alcoholism could run in families. A tendency to see a little harmless drinking as "alcoholism" could run in those families too. And that's what was happening here. I could feel it coming.

"Now, I've looked into the Betty Ford Clinic…" my dad began.

And there it was. I was being labeled as an alcoholic. Just what I wanted first thing in the morning, before my second cup of coffee, after a night with no dinner and not nearly enough wine.

"It's expensive," Dad was saying, "but I'm willing to pay for it, if it will help you. I think you do need help. Of course, that's just my opinion." He looked up at me for some kind of response but in my head I'd already left the room.

I let an uncomfortable pause linger in the air. And then I said, coldly, "I'm going to get one more cup of coffee before we leave." There was no way I was going to the Betty Ford Clinic. I didn't even want to talk about drinking with my dad. It was a very uncomfortable subject. He could keep me from drinking in his house, but he couldn't make me talk about this.

I poured the cup of coffee, then simply turned and walked out the door, flatly ignoring everything he'd said. I didn't know what my dad made of it. And I didn't care. As far as I was concerned, the subject of my drinking was closed.

12

Lost Hours

DURING THE FIRST TEN YEARS OF MY DRINKING, I DROVE alone most of the time when I went to bars. It's said that God protects fools and drunks. And I was a fool to drive drunk. But for some reason, God protected me — yet everyone else within the range of my headlights was in danger.

When I first started drinking, I thought drunk driving wasn't a big deal. In those days, when people got caught for driving drunk, not much happened to them, as long as there was no accident and no one had gotten hurt. They might get a ticket, but more likely they'd get what we called "a slap on the wrist" — a stern warning from a police officer — and sent on their way. An exceptionally conscientious policeman might tail a person all the way home, but that was about it.

Today, driving under the influence is considered a serious offense. In California, it can get you ninety-six hours in jail, a suspended license and a fine. Some states even require that the driver attend a treatment program after their second citation. But when I was driving drunk, it was much more tolerated. And if no one was going to arrest me or slap me with a fine, I didn't see a problem as long as I could get home intact.

Looking back on it now, I realize that I could easily have killed someone by driving drunk. But that didn't even occur to me for years.

* * *

Many mornings I'd get up, hung over, and sit in my bedroom with the radio on, drinking my morning coffee. I'd try to remember driving home the night before. Wracking my brain, I'd try to picture the road up ahead or see myself making a turn at the corner. But nothing came to mind. How could I have no memory at all of driving home?

Since it happened so often, I got into the habit of lifting up the curtains first thing in the morning to see if my car was outside. I was afraid of looking out to see my parking spot empty and not being able to remember where I'd left my car. But it scared me even more to see my car parked in my parking spot, then have no recollection at all of getting home.

Sometimes, I'd wonder if it were possible that someone else had driven me home. But I couldn't remember that either. Over the years, I asked Julie how I'd gotten home so many times that it was like a running joke between us.

Sometimes I'd have to ask Julie, "Do you know how I got home last night?"

"What are you talking about?" she'd say. "You drove yourself home. Don't you remember? You knocked on the door around two thirty in the morning. I opened it and you walked in, laughing, and saying you couldn't find your keys."

"What happened to my keys?"

"They were in your hand."

Julie would describe the things I did and said before I staggered off to bed. It was like hearing about someone else's life. I wouldn't remember it at all. In fact, I usually couldn't remember anything after eight or so the previous night.

No matter how many times it happened, it always shocked me. I knew the bars I'd ended up at before then. That was it. I could've gone anywhere after that and, for all I knew, I did.

Those lost hours haunted me, but the idea of not drinking was even worse, so I put up with it. If it started to worry me too much, I'd call a taxi to take me to the bars. This seemed like a perfect solution. If I didn't bring my car, I couldn't drive it home. Problem solved.

* * *

Not far from my house were three sleazy bars within three blocks of each other. Two of them were close together, but the third was further away.

Before I left home, I'd take about fifty dollars for drinks and cabs. It was easy to burn through fifty dollars in a night. From the apartment, I'd call a taxi to take me to the first bar. Then, once I was drunk, I'd start feeling restless and wonder what was going on at the other bars. It seemed to me that I might be missing a better time elsewhere. So I'd walk the two blocks to the second bar, so I could see what the people there were up to and party with some new faces. Since the other two bars were closer together, I'd walk back and forth between the three bars for hours.

Afterward, if I got hungry, I'd call a second taxi to take me downtown to the only restaurant open twenty-four hours a day, so I could eat my regular order — a patty melt. I always ordered a patty melt.

If I didn't eat a little food before coming home I'd often be so drunk that when the taxi pulled into my driveway I'd just hop out and stumble upstairs to the apartment, "forgetting" to pay the taxi driver.

Looking for my keys seemed to require such extraordinary effort. If I did manage, by some fluke, to find the keys in my purse, there was no way that I could find the right key and fit it into that ridiculously tiny slot in the lock. So I gave that up very quickly. I knew if I had any problems getting into my apartment, I could call out to Julie and she'd crawl out of bed to rescue me.

Most of the time, the taxi drivers resigned themselves to not getting paid and drove off, cursing me. But once, a driver came after me. Apparently, he'd let it go a few times and wasn't going to take it anymore. After I'd stumbled into the house, he shut off his engine, stomped up our stairs and knocked on the door.

By then, I'd already fallen into bed with all my clothes on and passed out. I never even heard him. Julie answered the door.

"Listen," the cabbie said angrily. "She didn't pay me again. I've put up with this too many times. This is how I make my living. I need to get paid. If you don't give me some money tonight, I'm calling the police."

"No problem," said Julie. "I'll be right back." She went in my room and took the money from my wallet to pay him.

* * *

One night when I was making my rounds between the three sleazy bars, I met a girl named Pam. She was a few years younger than I and not very attractive. In the whole time we knew each other, I never saw her drunk. She'd call me up and say, "Why don't you meet me at the bar tonight after work? I'll buy you a drink." When I arrived, she'd be sitting at the bar, chain smoking cigarettes and nursing a drink that would last for hours.

These bars were truly sleazy but I liked going to them. For one thing, Pam and I were often the youngest people there. And it seemed clear to me that I was usually one of the most attractive. It didn't make a lot of difference anyway because the regulars were hard drinkers who started early and devoted their days to drinking. At any given time, most of the customers at the bar were drunk. I liked the attention I got from both the men and women. Men paid attention to me because I was younger and prettier than the other women in the bar. Many of the women took me under their wings and treated me like a daughter. Either way, I got a lot attention in the sleazy bars. I didn't have the competition that I would have in the trendy bars.

I'd usually get to the bars just after lunch, around two. Even though I'd sometimes gone to bed drunk the night before and spent the bulk of the morning nursing a hangover before coming back to the bars, I felt sorry for these pathetic losers who had nothing to do but drink every day. If they were drunk by the time I got here, what time had they started drinking? I wondered. How sad.

* * *

Drinking was a calculated affair. If I were going out alone, I'd have the driving situation to work out. Should I drive myself and try to remember where I parked my car or should I take a series of cabs? If I had plans to go out on a date, it was much easier to manage. I'd make sure to set things up as inconspicuously as possible, so that my date would have to drive me home.

Most of the time I'd find some excuse to explain why I'd rather be picked up than meet the guy at a restaurant. If I didn't know him well, I'd usually say, "My car has been acting up lately. Would you mind picking me up? I'll buy you a drink!"

"No problem," the guy would say. Half the time, he'd add, "You don't need to buy me a drink." Even better! That little conversation was like a gift of freedom to me. It meant I could enjoy a long, private happy hour before going out, which was one of my favorite things.

But first I had to evaluate my timeline so I could execute my drinking calculations. What time was I going to be picked up? How long did I have until then? How many drinks were in the fridge? The goal was to try to figure out what time I could start my afternoon drinking, so I could finish all the beer in the house just in time to be picked up.

Nothing was worse than finishing early and having to

wait alone in the house — with nothing to drink! I couldn't let that happen. Making a correct calculation was essential.

My natural drinking speed — unhurried, at a normal pace — was about one beer every thirty minutes. Two beers an hour.

So it was simple math. Suppose some guy was going to pick me up at 6:00 P.M. and all I had in the house was a six-pack. (Disappointing, but okay.) Here's the equation:

$$6 \text{ cans of beer} \div 2 \text{ beers/hour} = 3 \text{ hours of drinking time}$$

That meant I could start around three in the afternoon. If I bided my time till around quarter past three or three-thirty, it would be ideal. That way, I'd be able to drink a little faster and be done right on schedule — a few minutes before six. (I liked to take the last five or ten minutes to brush my teeth thoroughly and put on lipstick before my date arrived.)

By that time I'd be buzzed, but not drunk. At first I convinced myself that I was doing all this so I'd be in a more gregarious frame of mind. It made me more fun on a date and helped me to relax and have a good time too. But the truth was that I was worried. I knew I'd only be able to have a few drinks on the date, so I felt more secure drinking ahead of time. Then I would be assured of having a nice buzz going for me throughout my entire date.

* * *

I loved my before-date drinking. In fact, sometimes the before-date drinking was more fun than the date itself.

To really enjoy myself, I needed music and noise. So I had my music playing the entire time. When Julie was at work, I loved it even more. With the whole apartment to myself, I could leave my bedroom door open and crank up the music.

Naturally, there were calculations involved in my

smoking too. If I smoked too much, my lungs felt tight, so smoking — and breathing — were less enjoyable. So I had to ration my cigarettes carefully.

Whenever I had my first drink of the day, I would smoke one cigarette. Then I'd wait for at least a half-hour before having my second one. I was always watching the clock. I had to hold off on that second cigarette for thirty minutes.

As soon as the clock hit twenty-nine minutes, I'd pick up the pack and get ready to light up another one. By that time, I'd been looking forward to it for twenty minutes. Nothing could've made me miss that moment. If the building had caught fire, I would've probably lit my cigarette before running out.

But once it was lit, I was very cool about it. You can easily get ten puffs from one cigarette. If you buy the longer brands, you can get even more. I made a practice of taking only about seven puffs, eight at the most, before stubbing it out. It was something I was proud of.

When I did that at a bar, people would say to me, "You're wasting so much of your cigarette. Why don't you smoke it down to the butt?"

The answer was easy: I was in control.

Some people are so addicted, so desperate for that little stick of nicotine that they have to suck everything they can out of it, but not me. I may have been addicted to cigarettes, but I wasn't that addicted, I told myself.

Stopping after seven or eight puffs was just a matter of self-respect. It didn't bother me. It showed who was in control. I knew exactly how many puffs I'd taken. Exactly how many cigarettes I'd had in the previous few hours. Exactly how many I'd have in the next thirty minutes too. Was nicotine controlling me? Was alcohol controlling me? What a ludicrous idea.

Observe: Seven puffs.

* * *

A few years before I stopped smoking altogether, I was flying back to California with Julie, after we'd visited our extended family in Michigan. Our airline reservations said that we'd have thirty minutes between flights in Chicago. Julie and I both were looking forward to our cigarettes during that layover.

What we didn't realize was that thirty minutes was barely long enough for us to cross the airport to catch our second flight. As soon as the first plane landed at the airport, we had to run for the next plane.

"If we hurry," Julie said, rushing down the terminal ahead of me, dragging her hand luggage behind her, "we can have a quick smoke before we board."

It was an exciting idea, but impossible. By the time we got to the gate, the other passengers were already getting on the plane.

"Chicago to Los Angeles?" the airline attendant said when she saw us. Panting for air, we nodded silently, in unison, and she waved us on board the plane. Julie and I exchanged a disappointed glance. Three more minutes and we could've had half a cigarette, maybe more. But there weren't three minutes to spare.

For the first hour or so, I was in a lousy mood. When I needed a cigarette, I became anxious and irritable. Now I was going to have to wait the entire flight before I could smoke.

"If you attempt to smoke in the restrooms," the smiling hostess said, "a smoke alarm will go off, alerting the captain."

"Great," I scowled.

"Have some plane food," Julie grinned, when the meal service came around, "You can choose from Chicken Surprise or Tuna Surprise. That should calm you down." For some reason, Julie seemed more comfortable than I did with not smoking for the duration of the flight. She was smoking a lot more than I was. I didn't understand it. Not having a cigarette for so long was all that I could think about for much of the flight. I thumbed through one identical flight magazine after another for a couple of hours and tried to think of something else, but now and then my hand would drift down to the pack of cigarettes sitting in my purse. There was nothing I could do but give them a pat and wait.

When we landed, I rushed off the plane and found an open spot in the airport to light up my cigarette. Taking that first drag felt like coming up for air from the bottom of the ocean. Smoking was so grand at that moment. I was happy again.

* * *

At my peak, I was smoking two packs. That's forty cigarettes — each and every day. After I quit drinking in 1987, the number of cigarettes dropped dramatically. Within a few years, I'd cut back to seven cigarettes a day, then four a day and, finally, to two a day.

I had a few reasons for cutting back.

The biggest reason was that I didn't want to feel beholden to cigarettes. The idea of not smoking scared me. I could barely entertain the thought. And deep inside, that bothered me. I gradually cut back because I couldn't stand to face my dependency full on. I was too scared to even think about quitting altogether. That's what a stronghold smoking had on me. I was addicted to cigarettes and didn't want to admit it.

* * *

The other thing I loved to do during my before-date drinking was to try on lots of clothes. Sometimes they were things I hadn't even worn. I'd go shopping for the fun of it, then drop the shopping bag on the floor of my closet or hang the clothes up, still inside their bags, and months would go by before I'd open those bags again. A lot of times, I didn't even remember what was in them. But that was fine because opening each bag was a surprise, like opening a present. It made my time getting ready for a date all the more enjoyable.

I had taken the bigger of the two bedrooms when Julie and I moved in. I had to pay more rent, but the room also had a vanity area with a big mirror and walk-in closet. Before a date, I spent lots of time looking in my mirror. Although I was still about thirty or forty pounds overweight during my drinking years, I looked quite attractive — especially if I sat down on my bed at just the right angle — so I could only see myself in the mirror from my head down to my chest. There was no denying it. The top third of my body looked great!

I'd hold my beer in one hand and my cigarette in the other, then I'd pose at different angles in front of the mirror while I lip-synced to the songs on the radio. I knew every little "ooh" and "oh, yeah" of the Top 40 songs they played.

Julie had a record player in her room. Sometimes I'd put on a favorite album — usually The Commodores or Barry Manilow — and drink my beer while I listened to the love songs. I'd get very emotional, thinking about a current or lost love. The more beer I'd had, the more emotional I would become.

If I were listening to the radio, I'd get all excited when a song came on by a female artist that I liked. That's when my lip-syncing turned into a full-blown performance. For a few minutes, my bedroom would disappear and I'd imagine myself singing to an audience, just as I'd done as a child, singing along to Cher.

I loved singing. It was easy to get totally lost in the fantasy, standing up on a stage before adoring fans, looking fantastic and singing these songs. My beer would transform into a mike and I'd pour my heart out in each song — glancing over, now and then, at the mirror, to reassure myself that I still looked great.

My goal was to be big and important someday. Maybe

I'd be a famous singer. Every time I sang along to the radio in my before-date drinking, it seemed obvious to me that my dreams would come true one day — whenever "one day" came along.

* * *

If all went well, by five thirty — before my date at six — I'd have one last beer left. But sometimes, when I checked the fridge, there wasn't one — there were two beers left. It gave me a kind of happy, giddy feeling. What a "good girl" I was.

"See? I don't have a drinking problem!" I'd scoff. It was perfectly obvious. I could have had every single one of those beers, but there were two beers left! That wasn't even part of the plan. I'd planned to drink more and I'd had less. Does an alcoholic do that? I think not.

It didn't happen often, but when it did, it was a moment of pride.

To celebrate, I'd drink both the beers.

By the time my date approached, I was so amenable that, if I happened to get a phone call from my date, saying he'd be late by an hour or so, it was no problem either. That type of emergency was something I could easily handle. There was a liquor store a block away. I'd just make my way over there and pick up another six-pack.

13

Guys, Guys, Guys!

JUST ABOUT EVERY TIME I WENT OUT DRINKING AND dancing, I met new men. At one of the dance clubs, there were a lot of Arab guys, some of the same ones I'd met before and some new ones.

They liked me because I had an "Arab look." Also, I was polite and attentive to them, which was important in the Arab community. Besides, I'd heard that Arab men felt free to express their anger if a woman did something to make them mad, and they could get mad at a woman over anything. So it only made sense for me to be courteous and low-key around them.

Even though it was against their religion to drink and go to bed with lots of women, they had so much money they could get almost any woman they dated into bed, after wining and dining her and treating her well.

I liked going out with them partly because they had a fantastic sense of humor. But I also knew that if we had an argument, I could leave and not be too bothered by the relationship ending. The cultural differences between us were so great that I felt safe. I assumed I'd never get close enough to them to be hurt if we broke up.

There were two guys in particular that I enjoyed talking to. I'd spend the evening at their table, letting them ply me with drinks, then get so drunk that I'd end up going home with one of them.

One morning I woke up with a pounding headache, alone in a king-size bed, having no memory of where I was. I could see it was a nice home I was in but I had no idea who it belonged to. I vaguely remembered partying with one of the Arab guys.

I got out of bed and saw I was wearing a long, flowing Arab gown. I had no recollection of how I happened to be wearing it. When I walked to the window, I looked down from the second floor onto the grounds of a beautiful estate with gardens and well-manicured lawns.

Walking into the hallway, I heard several voices, talking and laughing in Farsi. I made my way toward them. It was a big, open kitchen with terra cotta floors. The sun was streaming in through the French doors, leading out to the lawn.

Mohammed looked over at me and gave me a big smile. "Good morning, Linda. Did you sleep well?"

And then I remembered. I'd left the club with him the night before. I didn't remember much else, but if I'd come home with him, it didn't take too much imagination to figure out what probably happened next.

Five other men were sitting around the kitchen table, drinking cups of coffee, smoking and talking. I had no idea who they all were. I was hung over, but I knew also that Arab men weren't supposed to drink alcohol. I didn't want to introduce myself by mentioning that I'd had too much to drink, although they all probably knew.

"Yes, I did. Is there any coffee?" I needed caffeine desperately.

"Yes, there is some made," Mohammed said, speaking in Farsi to a young guy standing out of the way. He poured me a cup of coffee and brought it over to me.

As I talked with Mohammed and his friends, I learned that this beautifully furnished home had been rented indefinitely by the Saudi Arabian government for Arab students and diplomats visiting Santa Barbara. It had six bedrooms, five baths and an enormous swimming pool. But there were cameras everywhere. The security was so tight that if someone came to the gate of the house they'd have to ring the bell and give their name at the gate. The guard at the gatehouse was posted twenty-four hours a day.

Whether they owned them or not, Saudi Arabian guys often lived in exquisite homes. Money was no object for them and that appealed to me. They had a way of making me feel special. Sometimes I fantasized about what my life would be like were I to marry one of them. I wouldn't have to work. I could live a life of luxury. It sounded so wonderful to me. But I knew I could never make it work. There were too many cultural differences, for one thing. But there was also another little problem ....

One of my favorite Arab guy friends was Ibrahim. We dated for only a short time, but when I went over to his house and we had several drinks he took me into the bedroom, threw me on the bed and we had sex.

Afterward, he asked me to take a shower with him. I weighed 185 then and couldn't have Ibrahim see me naked. Sex was different. I'd always have the lights off so the man couldn't see my body. Ibrahim insisted I take off my clothes and shower with him. We got into a shouting match because I wasn't about to take off my clothes, and I never dated him again.

I didn't really care all that much when the Arab boyfriends didn't work out. They all seemed to want to control me and I wouldn't let them. When I drank heavily, I tended to yell and scream and get into fights with my boyfriends. Most Arab guys I knew would never have put up with that. But I found lots of other guys who were more than willing.

* * *

Jack was a good example. Although I went out with a lot of different guys when I was drinking, not many of them could be called a "relationship." My relationship with Jack lasted six months. It was the shortest relationship I'd ever been in. Since he was about three years younger than I, he also had the distinction of being the youngest man I ever dated. And now that I think of it, he was, at 6'5", probably the tallest guy I'd ever been out with as well. But the marvels pretty much end there.

Jack was literally the guy next door — a carpet cleaner. One night, we ended up talking in the parking lot of our apartment complex. The next day, there was a note on my car from Jack saying what a good time he had had talking with me. He said he'd like to ask me out sometime.

I was excited to have such a good-looking man take an interest in me. Before long, we were dating regularly. But I saw quickly that, although he was a nice guy, he was passive. So I never had much respect for him.

Without even trying, I easily took control of the relationship. I didn't like it. I always wanted him to be able to stand up and take control in situations, but he never did. So I settled for the fact that he was company and didn't seem to mind my drinking. But in the back of my mind I was always open to another man if someone I liked more came along.

One particular night I'd been drinking for several hours when I told Jack I wanted to go get Mexican food. It was one of the few foods that seemed to be able to soak up the alcohol in my system and make me more alert, even if I were drunk. Jack loved Mexican food, so he happily agreed. We went to a little place around the corner called La Casa. With its simple food and nonstop Mexican music in the background, it was popular with the locals.

When the waiter came around to take our drink orders, I said, "I'll take a lite beer." "I'll have the same," Jack said.

As the waiter left to get the drinks, Jack looked around at everyone drinking Margaritas and said to me, "Oh, I should have gotten a Margarita!"

"Just get up and go tell the waiter you've changed your mind and you want a Margarita instead," I insisted.

"No. I already placed my order. I don't want to make things hard on the waiter."

I was not quite drunk yet, but I was working on it. And it seemed to me that this was the perfect time to speak my mind about how I hated Jack's passiveness. The more I thought about it, the more worked up I got. I would not live my life with a passive man anymore. I hated to see people live like that — never asking for what they wanted, never speaking up. Why couldn't he be more assertive?

I launched into a tirade that lasted over the next several drinks. Listening to me tell him how to live his life, Jack politely drank his lite beer when the waiter brought it. Then he started ordering Margaritas. After we'd both had a few more drinks, I leaned over the table and whispered to Jack that I wanted to go home and hop into bed with him after dinner.

He looked at me coldly. "We'll have sex another time when you're not drunk." He had the idea that we should just eat when the food arrived, then I could go home to my own bed.

Always feeling amorous when I drank, I resented the fact that he wouldn't sleep with me. I ordered another beer. I'd had about six beers at the restaurant by the time Jack told me to stop drinking. After hours of drinking at home all afternoon plus those six beers, I was drunk.

The dinner came and we ate. I could only eat a little because I'd drunk so much. It was common for me to take most of my food home when I went to restaurants. As long as I had beer in front of me, I wasn't hungry.

During dinner I started getting mean to Jack, trying to pick a fight with him. I went back to my theme about how he was so passive it made me think less of him as a man, then I asked him why he couldn't stand up for himself. Still simmering over the fact that he'd implied I wasn't attractive when I was drunk, I threw in the idea that I thought passive men weren't sexy.

Jack leaned over the table and spoke softly, so only I

could hear him. "I don't take control when we're together because YOU always have to be in control. Everything has to be Linda's way or not at all. You're always controlling everything in our relationship — where we go to dinner, what time we go to bed, what bars and restaurants we go to, what I can do when I'm not with you. You hate me being passive? Well, I hate you being controlling!" Sulking, he went back to drinking his beer.

I couldn't believe how rude he'd been to me! I ordered another beer and, even though he'd insisted I stop, Jack didn't say a word. But when the waiter brought me my beer, Jack stopped me and said, "If you order any more beer, I'm leaving."

Normally, I wouldn't have believed he'd leave, but this time I did. I leaned over the table and said, quietly, "Shut up. Don't threaten me. People are staring at you." I was slurring my words quite a bit at this point.

"Me? They're staring at me? They're staring at YOU, because you're drunk!"

And they were. When I was drunk, my voice got loud. And I was usually oblivious of people looking at me. I told Jack I was going to the bathroom and almost fell over getting out of my chair. On the way, I stopped by the bar and told the bartender to send a lite beer to my table and put it on the tab. Then I went to the bathroom and had a drunken chuckle.

The beer was sitting on the table when I got back.

"Did you order this?" Jack snapped at me.

"Of course not. I went to the bathroom like I told you."

He didn't say anything. But when the bill came, he asked me to pay for some of it, since most of the bill was for my beers.

This made me angry. I was already feeling argumentative and now he was just making it worse. "You're the guy! You should pay for me. I want a man who takes care of his woman. If you love me, you'll pay."

Then I tried to get up from my chair to make a dramatic exit, but somehow I managed to kick its leg as I got up. The chair fell in front of me and I went tumbling over the top of it, landing flat on the floor. My knee hurt. I'd dropped my purse. And I was having a lot of trouble disentangling myself from the damn chair, when Jack came over to help me get up.

I started yelling at him. We had an audience, but I didn't care. I was so lost in my drunkenness that I barely knew what I was doing. I started crying and Jack literally lifted me up off the floor. I have no memory of it, but he must have paid the bill. The next thing I knew, he was helping me out of his car and into my apartment. Julie was home so she helped me into bed.

Clearly, my whole assertiveness conversation had backfired. Even though I had wanted to see Jack be more assertive while I dated him, I certainly didn't want that to impinge on my drinking!

The next day was Friday. I was hung over and stayed to myself all day. If Jack had called, I would have talked to him. But he didn't call. He did call on Saturday, though, to see how I was feeling. He told me he was sorry about how things had worked out the night we went out to the restaurant. And he asked me not to drink so much any more.

Then something happened on Sunday. When I woke up that morning, I just didn't want to be Jack's girlfriend any more.

It was the strangest thing — how my feelings for him just seemed to evaporate overnight. On Thursday, I'd hated the idea of him leaving me in the restaurant. On Friday, I missed him terribly. On Saturday, I'd felt relieved that things were going to be better between us. But on Sunday, I knew it was over.

It had nothing to do with the fact that he'd asked me not to drink so much any more. Even though I hated that more than anything, I was sure I wasn't choosing drinking over love. That would be ridiculous. It was just something about Jack, apparently. He wasn't really the one for me. That must be it.

I called Jack that Sunday and told him I had to come over to talk to him. When I walked in, I sat down on the chair next to the couch where he was sitting and said to him, "Jack, I think we need to break up. I like you, and we can still be friends, but we have to break up."

"Okay," he said.

I couldn't believe how easy it was. I'd been trying to think up reasons in case he asked me anguished questions about why we had to break up, hadn't he meant anything to me, etc., but no. I didn't get any resistance at all. He was happy to go along.

And I was in high spirits. I got up and said, "Okay. Well! Talk to you later then."

"Okay," he said again and hugged me goodbye.

14

More Broken Promises

As usual, I wasn't alone for long. Russell, the landscaper at the apartments where Julie and I lived struck up a pleasant conversation with me one day outside our apartment.

About a week later I ran into him while I was shopping at the mall. He asked if he could stop by my apartment the next time he was at my complex working. That way we'd have more time to talk.

"Sure," I said. "Come by whenever you'd like. We can have a few drinks."

Russell smiled and I noticed what a great smile he had. "I do like a beer or two sometimes," he said.

"Great. I'll go buy some beer and have it ready for when you come."

When he came by the next week, we drank and talked and had a really enjoyable time. We ended up dating for about a year.

For his birthday, I made a decorative gift certificate for dinner and drinks at any restaurant of his choosing. Like Jack, Russell loved Margaritas. So he decided he wanted to go to El Gato, a Mexican restaurant downtown. I was glad. I loved their Margaritas too.

Normally, Russell wasn't a big drinker, but on this particular night he wanted to be able to drink and not worry about either one of us driving, so he offered to pay for the cab rides to and from the restaurant, which was only about two miles from my apartment. I was all for that.

We got to the restaurant about three in the afternoon. I started drinking beer and Russell drank Margaritas. When I saw Russell getting buzzed, I enjoyed it, because he seldom got buzzed with me. He had always been a little too reserved. Margaritas helped him relax and have a good time. It looked like we were going to have a night to remember.

When the waiter came to our table, I told him we would be having an extended happy hour to celebrate Russell's birthday. It wasn't busy in the restaurant, so we didn't feel as if we were holding up a table drinking.

The waiter was fine with it. "You just let me know when you'd like to order," he said.

I was glad to have a cool, understanding waiter. I'd have to remember to leave him a generous tip.

As the afternoon wore on, we drank quite a bit. I drank much more than Russell did, of course. I even ordered a few Mexican beers on tap after I'd had several lite beers. I was feeling high.

Around five, the waiter asked us if we'd like to order.

"No, we're fine!" I said, articulating every word as carefully as I could. "Just bring us another round."

"Come on, Spunk!" Russell said, using his nickname for me. "Why don't we get something to eat now? I'm hungry."

"No. I'm not hungry yet. I'm finally having fun with you." I knew when I did eat, it would bring me down from my high. "Eat some chips, if you're hungry."

"I want some real food."

"It's my birthday present to you. Let's have one more drink," I said, really feeling the beer now, since I'd drunk all the beers so quickly on an empty stomach. And then I leaned against him affectionately. "I'm so glad you'll be spending the night with me tonight," I added, hoping he'd be more inclined to let me have my way. It was usually easy to manipulate Russell with sex. If I offered it, I could get away with murder. But when I was in a bad mood, I withheld it. He fell for it every time.

"Okay," he said, giving in. "But I gotta eat soon..."

All right! That meant I'd get to have at least one more beer before dinner.

We had another round of drinks, then placed our orders for food. It was around seven o'clock by then, but I wasn't hungry, so I only ate a little bit and took the rest of my meal home, as usual. By eight o'clock, we had finished eating and drinking. I was paying for everything and figured it would be about thirty dollars. But when I reached for the bill, I saw that the bar bill alone was forty-two dollars. The total for food and drinks was fifty-five dollars plus the large tip which would be at least ten dollars! I wasn't working and that was a lot of money to me.

"Oh, no, Russell. Look at how much this is!" I said loudly, and panicking. "It must be wrong! We didn't drink this much. It can't be right! Russell, ask the waiter, Okay? Oh NO!!"

Russell tried to calm me down and finally agreed to pay his share, so I could cover my own part. I let him pay and stopped shouting. The next day, Russell said I had been somewhat coherent, but I'd been so loud, complaining about the bill, that everyone in the room had been staring at us. It was embarrassing for Russell. I would've been embarrassed too had I known what a scene I was causing, but I couldn't remember a thing.

* * *

Like many of my boyfriends, Russell began to ask me not to drink. One Saturday, we were going to have dinner together at Paul and Jenny's house and he begged me not to drink before we went. Paul and Jenny were close friends of Russell's whom he knew for a long time. From everything he'd said about them, they sounded like enjoyable people. He was eager for us to meet.

Russell had to work all day, but he called me in the afternoon to see what I was up to. (This was basically code for "Have you been drinking?") Well, I had been drinking, naturally, but I told him I'd been out shopping. I said I was going to be home for the next few hours cleaning until I met him to go to Paul and Jenny's house.

It was not entirely a lie. I hadn't gone shopping, but I had been cleaning at home. I'd just been drinking beer while I was cleaning. I'd bought a six-pack that morning for the long afternoon. Having worked out my beer schedule, I knew I could drink one beer an hour and not be drunk when I went to dinner that night. I might even be able to hide it from Russell. Or, if worse came to worse, I could say I'd just had a quick beer after I'd gotten back to the house. Half a beer even. Nothing to speak of.

Well, that was the plan, anyway. In reality, I ended up drinking the whole six-pack in about four hours. I did a half-hearted job of cleaning the apartment and actually spent most of the afternoon drinking and playing albums. (If I didn't feel like singing, I'd play Barry Manilow and pretend that every love song Barry sang referred to Russell).

I'd take breaks from cleaning and sit on the bed with my beer and cigarette and think about what Barry Manilow was telling me about Russell — how he loved me and wanted to be with me forever. I got so much more romantic when I was drinking, that by the end, I was feeling turned on toward Russell.

Because I'd finished most of the beer early, I still had two hours to kill before leaving and I got myself into a predicament. I was truly buzzed by the time I had one drink left. I tried my best to nurse it and make it last, because I shouldn't drive the two miles to Russell's house when I was buzzed like this. I knew I could get arrested.

But, of course, it was only two miles through a residential neighborhood. So I decided I'd just have to risk it. If I told Russell I couldn't come to dinner because I'd been drinking all day, he'd tell me not to come over that night at all. And after Barry Manilow, I really wanted to see him and have a good time.

I made it over to Russell's house without being stopped. I'd squirted a little perfume on and brushed my teeth and tongue, so he wouldn't smell the beer. And then, for good measure, I promised myself that that would be the last time I would drive after drinking.

I couldn't keep chancing it. Even when I was buzzed, it scared me to think that I'd taken such a chance by driving.

I walked up to Russell's door, knocked and walked in as I always did.

Russell came over to give me a hug. Then he pulled back and looked me in the eye, trying to see if I'd been drinking.

I quickly looked away. "Are you ready to go?" I asked, being careful not to slur my words. I thought the sentence sounded pretty good. He shouldn't be able to detect any slurring.

"Were you drinking, Spunk?" I knew he could see by my eyes I was buzzed.

I couldn't lie. "Nothing much. I had two beers all afternoon," I lied. I tried convincing Russell to just let it go, so we could head over to Paul and Jenny's.

He was disappointed in me. He said we could go to dinner. "But, please, please don't drink much tonight. One or two beers at the most!"

Since my promises meant nothing, I happily agreed.

Paul and Jenny, to my surprise, had some homemade beer that they had literally made in their bathtub. "Drink as much as you like!" they laughed. They were proud of their beer.

We had a barbeque, then laughed and talked afterwards. Paul was getting drunk and I just kept drinking that homemade beer. I was getting extremely drunk and slurring my words.

When Russell tried to get me to stop drinking, Paul

kept saying, "Leave Linda alone, man! She's enjoying herself." I really liked this guy.

Around eleven o'clock, I was almost falling-over drunk.

Russell took my cup of beer away from me. I started to run after him, saying, "Give me back my beer!" I was fuming! I was unbelievably drunk, but I couldn't stop drinking... not just yet.

Russell had evaded me. So I picked up his beer glass and went around the side of the house to drink it with my cigarette.

In a few minutes, Russell found me. "You've ruined this get-together," he said. "Because you're drunk. Didn't I ask you not to drink?"

When Paul and Jenny came over to see what we were doing, Russell said we were leaving. But I hit his arm and disagreed. Russell gave me a look, then excused himself and went back to his apartment. "I'll come back when you've calmed down," he said.

I was glad to see him leave. Now I could party with Paul and Jenny.

When the coast was clear, Paul leaned over and whispered, "Russell's gone. Do you want another beer?"

The homemade beer was hitting me twice as fast as my usual lite beers, but I gladly followed Paul to the kitchen anyway. I knew I was almost to the point where I couldn't drink anymore, but I decided to keep going as long as I could.

Paul, Jenny and I sat on their front lawn. It was late. We sat and talked for what seemed like hours. I just kept drinking until I finally passed out on the lawn.

Apparently Paul went to get Russell, because he couldn't get me to wake up. Then Russell and Paul carried me back to Russell's house and they put me in the bed.

The next day Russell was quiet when I got up. He said firmly, "I don't want to see you anymore if you intend to keep drinking. After that performance last night, I will never allow myself to get in that situation with you again, is that understood?"

I didn't say much because I had a terrific hangover. Russell drove me home in silence on his way to work. When he dropped me off he said he needed a few days to think. He said I shouldn't call him, but he'd call me when he was ready. When a guy said that, it always put fear into me, because no matter what I didn't want to be alone.

Things were never the same between us again.

* * *

A few months before Russell and I broke up, I met Steve, who was soon to become one of the most important men in my life.

Steve was a bartender at a local bar that my sister Julie and I hung out at. And he asked me if I wouldn't mind going to dinner with him some night to discuss Julie. He claimed to be infatuated with her, not me.

Since I was still dating Russell, I asked him what he thought of me going out with Steve. Russell had met Steve at the bar too and he liked him.

"I think you should go, Spunk. Steve needs someone to talk to."

When Steve and I went out, he took me to a popular restaurant in town. We had to wait two hours to be seated, so naturally we drank for two hours. I was pretty buzzed when Steve just leaned over and kissed me in the bar. I was so excited. I felt feelings I hadn't felt in a long time. I realized I liked Steve…

For about two months I dated both Russell and Steve, until I realized my heart was with Steve and I'd have to tell Russell. At the time, Russell's thirty-three-year-old brother was dying of kidney failure from drinking. So it was difficult to break up with him. I felt badly about it. But leading him on was no better, so I told him I wanted to end it.

A week or so later, when his brother died, Russell called and asked me to spend the night with him. He was upset and said he really needed me to be with him.

Unfortunately, I had been drinking at home all afternoon. And, since we'd broken up, I was honest with him about it.

"I don't care," he said, his voice trembling slightly. "I really need you, Linda. Come on over. I'll pay for the cab."

When I got there, we lay down on the bed together and he started kissing me, wanting to have sex. "I'm in such pain," he said. "I need to feel your love."

"I'm sorry, Russell. I can't. I'm dating Steve now."

He was disappointed and turned his back to me in bed. We went to sleep together. When we got up early the next morning, he wouldn't say a word to me. He politely drove me home and when he dropped me off, he said, "I never want to see you or talk to you again."

I felt sad, but that was how it ended.

15

Dating the Bartender

FOR AN ALCOHOLIC, A BARTENDER IS A DREAM BOYFRIEND.
Steve was a bartender at one of my favorite bars. Once we started seeing each other regularly, the advantages were apparent right away. I liked going to visit Steve at the bar for a few reasons.

First of all, Steve was well-liked in his bar. When the regulars came in, he'd introduce me as his girl and they automatically liked me right away. How not? I was dating their favorite bartender! It gave me instant status at that bar.

Before long, I got to know most of the regulars by name. They'd come in, have a drink or two and sometimes sit there all day, getting drunk. Most were retired, but a lot of the young regulars came by every day too. They were just as happy to see me as I was to see them. It was like inheriting a new group of old friends.

The other thing I liked was that Steve would always give me at least one free drink when I came to the bar — sometimes even more. If I bought three beers, I'd pay for two. If I bought five, I'd pay for three. If I bought seven, I'd pay for four. Sometimes I did even better than that. One of the regulars might tell Steve to add my tab to theirs, so I wouldn't have to pay anything at all.

When I was ready to leave, I used to like to call Steve over to me and whisper, "Oh no! I don't have any money for a tip. How am I ever going to tip you?"

"We'll have to think of something," he'd purr in my ear and I'd smile.

He also liked it when I let him know I'd be available later. That alone could get me free drinks from Steve.

When I look back on it now I realize that, of all the boyfriends I ever had, Steve was the one who meant the most to me. I really respected him a lot. He was kind to everyone. People used to come up to me and say, "Linda, you've got yourself one of the good ones!" I was proud to be his girlfriend.

The first night my dad and his wife met him, they said, "Steve really loves you, Linda. Do you see how he looks at you?"

I knew he loved me and I loved him. And it wasn't just romantic love. Unlike some of the other guys I dated over the years, he truly cared about my well-being. He even tried to help me lose weight. He worked out regularly and was always encouraging me to work out too. I didn't do it at the time, but years later when I did start going to the gym I remembered some of the things he said about exercising and it really helped. We were good together. There were many things I loved about him. I still consider him the love of my life.

But the free beers didn't hurt!

*   *   *

One night when we were first dating, my mom called to say that she had season tickets for the symphony, but she wasn't going to be able to make it on a particular night. She wondered if Steve and I would like to go.

Steve and I were both excited about the idea of spending a glamorous night out on the town. Two months before the concert, he arranged for a co-worker to come in early to relieve him, so we could go. We made reservations at an elegant restaurant near the theatre so we could eat dinner beforehand.

Ordinarily, I didn't like planning events ahead of time. It interfered with my drinking regimen. And planning a meal immediately before a concert would mean hours and hours of nighttime without enough alcohol to make me high.

For some reason, I'd accepted the symphony tickets from my mom. I was so excited about spending the evening at the symphony with Steve, that I pushed aside my reluctance and made a plan.

We hadn't been dating long, but Steve was just starting to realize that my drinking could interfere with our lives, if he let it. So he made me promise that I'd have no more than three beers on the day of the symphony. Normally, there was no way I'd agree to that, but this time, to placate Steve, I laughingly agreed.

By the day of the symphony, my resistance had come back in full force. Why should I be restrained from drinking? This was my day, like any other, was it not? I should be able to do as I pleased. Having tickets to something later shouldn't deter me.

About two in the afternoon, I headed down to the bar to have a few drinks and see Steve. He was glad to see me, as always. We talked about how much we were looking forward to the symphony that night. But an hour or two later, Steve told me it was time for me to go. I'd had my three beers. The plan was that I would leave the bar — and not drink any more all day — until we met for dinner.

"What are you up to this afternoon?" Steve asked, innocently drying a glass at the bar.

"Oh, I don't know..." I lied.

I knew exactly what I was going to do. I was going to go to the liquor store and pick up a six-pack.

Steve must've sensed something, because he said, "You're not going to drink, are you?"

I picked up my purse and headed toward the door, blowing him a kiss at the last minute. "No. Call me later!" I had to leave fast, so he'd stop asking me questions.

I still had two perfectly good hours left to drink before I had to meet Steve back at the bar. Why should I sit home doing nothing, when I could be enjoying myself for those two hours? I knew Julie would be home that afternoon, so I bought some beer for her too. After sitting in the living room, drinking with Julie, I started to feel great and no longer wanted to go out that night.

"Why are we going to that stupid symphony?" I complained to Julie.

"You and Steve never go to cultural events. You'll enjoy it," she said.

That was easy for her to say. She didn't have to go. She didn't have any plans. She could sit at home drinking all night, then crawl into bed — exactly what I wanted to do. Reluctantly, I got up off the couch and went to my room to get dressed.

When we'd gotten the tickets, Steve and I had decided to go all out for this night. He was going to wear his black suit that looked so great on him. I would wear the only nice dress I owned — a black wool and crepe dress. I had told myself I'd lose a little weight before the big night, but I'd gained a few pounds instead. Luckily, I'd be wearing a black coat over my dress, so I wasn't concerned. Originally, I'd been planning to go the whole way and put my hair up. But things were looking different to me now.

I was on a roll. I had had three beers at the bar, then three more beers in those two hours at home. There was no way I was going to stop drinking now and I couldn't have stayed awake for the whole symphony anyway. Drinking a lot always made me sleepy earlier.

We'd have to go another time. Steve wouldn't like it, but what could he do?

I looked in the mirror at the dress. It did look pretty sensational on me, I had to admit. So I'd just wear it to something else another time. I drove to the bar to break the news to Steve in person. I figured, looking good in my fancy evening dress might help, so I left it on. Dress or no dress, I should have never gotten behind the wheel of a car after drinking six beers.

"I can't drive after four beers," I used to tell the regulars at the bar. "But after seven beers, I'm the best driver you've ever seen. I stay on the right side of the line. I dodge oncoming traffic. It's amazing. Everything's perfectly clear. It's like I have all the confidence in the world."

Twisted logic, but that's what I believed at the time. So I hopped into my car, one beer shy of my magic seven beers.

When I walked into the bar, there was an instant party atmosphere. Some of my favorite regulars were in the bar. I smiled and went over to greet everybody.

"Oooh! Look at this!" they said, when I came in, making a fuss over me in my fancy dress.

Right away, Coach called out to Steve, "I'd like to get Linda a drink!"

"No, she can't drink, Coach. We're going to dinner and the symphony," Steve said.

With a nod to Coach, I made my way over to Steve. I grabbed hold of his collar and pulled him toward me, so I could whisper in his ear. I was careful not to slur my words, but it took a lot of effort. "You know what? I really don't want to go to dinner before the symphony..."

Steve pulled back and looked at me. "You drank this afternoon, didn't you?" He was upset.

"No, no!" I lied. "I'm just saying, I'd rather stay here for a few drinks with you than go to dinner. I'm not hungry."

"I have reservations at that French restaurant downtown," Steve said. "I'd really like to keep them. We've been planning on this for two months now, Linda. I was very excited about going!" Steve looked crestfallen.

"Hey, it's no big deal," I said, trying to blow it off. "We'll go for French food some other time. But they're free symphony tickets. Let's stay here and sit together and talk for awhile, then we'll go hear the music."

"Are you sure you're not buzzed?" He looked directly into my eyes.

"No. I told you. Now, come on. I want a beer. We still have two hours."

After about thirty minutes, Steve went home to shower and grab a light dinner. I told him I'd eaten something earlier and wasn't hungry, which was a lie. If I didn't eat, I'd gradually get higher and higher. And that was the part I liked best.

After Steve left, I had several more beers. I was having a great time that night, moving from stool to stool, talking to all of my "friends."

Steve showed up right before seven thirty to pick me up, but by that time, I didn't want to go at all. I was feeling happy, and I was too drunk to enjoy a symphony. But I remembered the look of disappointment on his face earlier and couldn't bear to see that again, so I went along. If he knew how drunk I was when we left for the concert, he didn't let on.

As we walked down the red carpeted aisle to our seats in the balcony, I handed the tickets to Steve. "We'd better have aisle seats," I told him. "Because I don't want to crawl over a bunch of people every time I have to go to the bathroom."

But we had no such luck. There were four seats between our seats and the aisle. We had to step over people getting in and I knew I'd have to step over people getting out. "Oh, great!" I muttered. "Now, everyone will get mad at me when I say, 'Excuse me, excuse me,' every time I have to go to the bathroom."

"You shouldn't have had so much beer," Steve said.

The symphony started and I sat there in my seat, so drunk the room was nearly swimming in front of me. My eyes just wanted to close. Careful not to fall asleep or let my head drop over, I gently rested my eyes.

After the orchestra had warmed up and started the first piece, I needed to go to the bathroom. It was much too soon for that, so I shifted around in my chair. "Think about something else," I told myself. It was ridiculous to go back out already. They'd just started playing. I crossed my legs and started fidgeting with my beaded purse.

The long, slow passages of Schumann were beautiful to listen to, but I found myself rapidly tapping my foot. If only I could go to the bathroom. Steve gave me a warning look, but I just closed my eyes again and tried to keep my mind on something other than my bladder, which felt like it was just about to burst.

Finally, after what felt like a half-hour, I couldn't wait any longer. If I don't go now, I thought, my bladder is going to burst. I've got to go NOW. Nature took hold of me and I was out of my chair without even thinking about it.

Steve gave me an irritated look, but pulled in his knees and let me out. Then I had three more people to get by. ("Excuse me. Excuse me. Excuse me…") I went as slowly as I could because, after everything I'd had to drink, I wasn't feeling too stable and I was worried about falling over on someone. But I took my purse with me, in case they had wine in the lobby.

On the way to the ladies' room, I peeked around the corner into the lobby and saw that they did have wine for sale. It cheered me up right away. I quickly went to the bathroom, then hurried back out to the wine table and ordered a glass of wine. This was much more like it.

With my glass of wine in hand, I struck up a conversation with one of the ushers, a guy named Jeff, in his early twenties. As we talked, for some reason, he started to remind me of my brother David. In my drunken stupor, I started telling Jeff all about David's car accident a few years before and saying how much I missed him.

I drank the first glass of wine fast, then ordered another. My system was literally flooded with alcohol. The more I talked, the more upset I became. At some point, Jeff excused himself, saying he had to go check on a curtain or door or something. And before I knew it, I was sitting in one of the plush, high-backed chairs in the lobby, bawling my eyes out.

With my glass of wine in one hand, tilted at a precarious angle, and my cigarette in the other, I just sat in the chair and sobbed. Black streaks of make-up were following the tears down my face. And I was making no effort to sob quietly. I was letting it rip.

I have no idea how many people were watching me cry, but when I was in a mindset like that, I was in my own little sad world. I kicked off my strappy shoes and wiggled my toes in my stockings.

Not once did it cross my mind that Steve might be sitting inside the theatre, wondering what on earth had happened to me, probably fuming, as he tried to decide whether to keeping listening to the music or come looking for me in case I'd gotten into trouble. Steve was ancient history. I was living in the moment. And in the moment, the only thing I wanted was another drink.

After I'd been sitting there, crying and smoking and drinking wine for awhile, I looked up to see Jeff, standing over me, smiling kindly. "You're missing the symphony, you know. Don't you want to go back to hear some of it?"

No, I didn't, as a matter of fact, but I had a better idea.

With Jeff's help, I struggled back up onto my feet. Then, holding my strappy shoes in my hand, I just walked out the front door of the theatre. I had no idea where I was going, but, as always, I was looking for a bar where maybe I could meet some friendly people and have a little drink … and I did!

16

Threatening Suicide

ONE AFTERNOON, I WAS DRUNK AND WANTED TO GO OUT and be with people. When I started drinking, it didn't much matter to me if I were alone or at a bar with people. But once I got drunk, I had to have people around. So unfortunately, whenever I made a total fool of myself, there were always plenty of witnesses.

On this particular night, the only bar within walking distance was a sleazy dive down the street. I literally stumbled over to it. Julie knew the bartender there. When she saw me stagger out the front door in a stupor, she called the bar and told Maria, the bartender, not to serve me because I was drunk. Maria agreed not to serve me, but once I arrived, she served me anyway.

I sat down at the counter and started talking to an old man who looked like he'd been drinking for years. He bought me a beer and Maria got it for me. I stayed sitting next to this old man for two reasons: He was nice to me and he bought me drinks. But as soon as someone more interesting came along, I moved on.

After awhile, I saw Mike sitting at a table across the room. He was a guy my sister had dated several months before. As I crossed over to his table, I almost fell into him.

"Hi, Mike. Remember me?" I said, slurring.

Mike was cross-eyed drunk. Somehow, he always seemed to be drunk and belligerent. He started swearing at me, telling me to get away from him. As far as I knew, I'd never done anything to him, so I didn't know why he'd treat me like that. I decided to taunt him for being such a jerk. So I sat down next to Mike and asked him if he'd buy me a drink. He raised his voice even louder, swore at me and told me to get the hell away from him.

Suddenly I started feeling like I was going to pass out, so I hopped up and headed out the door. I hadn't paid for anything while at the bar. I don't know if I owed any money or not. I didn't say goodbye to anyone. I just left.

It was dark outside and I was so drunk that I didn't know where I was. I just turned left and started walking. My apartment was about a block away, but I couldn't figure out where it was, so I didn't get there right away.

Steve, in the meantime, had called the house, looking for me. Julie told him I had left for the bar, drunk, and had been gone for hours. Steve was worried because he knew how I was when I got drunk, so he got in his car and headed for the bar. On the way, he saw me stumbling along the overpass of the freeway in the dark. Afraid I'd lose my balance and fall over the edge, he drove up to me quickly and jumped out of the car.

He called out my name and I started yelling at him to leave me alone. I don't know why. Then I turned and kept walking away. (I always tried to get away from the boyfriends when I was drunk.) Running over to me, he started talking softly, trying to convince me to come home with him. When that didn't work, he picked me up, while I was kicking him, and threw me in his car. I was sobbing and screaming at him, but he just ignored me and kept driving me back to the house. As soon as my crying died down, I passed out.

At the time, I believed that Steve was the only man I ever really loved. It was such a detriment to my relationship with Steve that I was drinking heavily all the time. No matter how much we tried, our relationship could never really work while I was drinking. Instead of accumulating memories of happy times we spent together, we collected memories of horrible fights and embarrassing scenes.

* * *

In the beginning of our relationship, Steve sometimes threatened to take his key away from me when I was drunk. I would go to his house while he was at work and sit drinking on the couch all day. He'd come home to find me drunk. It was upsetting to him.

One night, he grabbed my keys from the table before I could reach them and took his key off of my key chain, then put my keys down. "I'm taking your key away from you for abusing the privilege," he said. "I asked you not to come over here and drink like this."

I tried arguing with Steve, but he told me he'd made the decision and he wasn't going to change his mind. Not having the keys to Steve's place meant I'd have to stay at my own place alone. The prospect of being alone terrified me.

I started crying and went into the bathroom. While I was thinking over arguments to use when I came back out, I opened the medicine cabinet to get some Tylenol for my headache. I was angry and frustrated and didn't care about anything. I just wanted to get back at Steve. So I thought, what the heck... and poured about twenty Tylenol into my hand.

I swallowed five at a time. After my first five, I started to cry again. I had no idea what twenty Tylenol would do to me. I was pretty sure I wouldn't die from it, but I was a little scared anyway. Still, my anger easily overpowered that fear. I knew Steve would save me. So I popped the twenty Tylenol and opened the bathroom door just a crack.

Steve had been watching TV and when a commercial came on, he pushed the bathroom door open to see what I was up to. I had carefully placed the half-empty Tylenol bottle in plain view, before sitting down on the edge of the bathtub.

"How many of these have you taken?" Steve demanded, holding the bottle up to me.

163

"I don't know. I'm going to kill myself." I said, then started crying hard.

Steve just stared at me and started reading the label on the bottle. I went over to lie on the bed, but fell asleep after a few minutes and slept through the night. When I woke up the next day, he had left for work. I started rummaging through every good hiding spot, looking for my key and finally found it. I put it back on my key chain and kept it. One way or another, I could usually win my arguments with Steve. Sometimes it took a day or so, but I usually got my way. And I wasn't above using extreme measures, if that was what it took.

* * *

When my brother David was killed in the car accident in 1983, my mother and father each got thirty thousand dollars from the driver's insurance company. My mom kept her thirty thousand dollars, but my dad said he didn't want any of it. So he decided to divide it between Craig, Julie and me.

Dad immediately gave ten thousand dollars to Craig. Julie and I assumed we'd be getting our money too. When a few months passed and there was no sign of the money, I asked my dad about it.

He said he thought that, while Julie and I were working at the Ming Tree, our lives were going nowhere. We were doing an easy job that didn't challenge us. He said the stipulation for getting the money was that we had to leave the motel. Julie and I liked working at the motel so we both figured we'd work there as long as we wanted, then collect the money, if and when we left.

But since we'd both lost our jobs at the Ming Tree we still hadn't gotten the money. Several days later, I called my dad. We chitchatted for a few minutes. Dad already knew Julie and I had lost our jobs. So with my heart pounding, I asked Dad if I could have my ten thousand dollars.

The tone of Dad's voice immediately changed. He began grilling me about my drinking.

"How many days has it been, Linda, since you had a drink?" He happened to ask at precisely the moment when I had stopped drinking for a few days. So, oddly enough, I could honestly say, "I haven't had a drink in five days. I feel wonderful."

Dad wasn't impressed with my five days of sobriety.

"No, I've decided to withhold the money from you girls right now. I just don't think it's the right time for either of you to get such a large sum of money."

"Craig got the money," I said a little more sternly. I was getting even madder, remembering that he'd only gotten this money because my brother had been killed.

"Craig got the money because he's going to get married and he needs it now."

"Well, we need the money because we don't have jobs anymore," I said sarcastically.

I knew it was useless talking anymore that day and we hung up. I related to Steve what my dad had said and then told him, "You know what? I'm going to go have a few drinks because I deserve it."

Steve asked me not to. I felt justified and was especially looking forward to drinking and commiserating with Julie about how unfair Dad was.

I went home, told Julie a little bit about the conversation with Dad, then asked her to join me for a few drinks. Julie was more than willing and we went out to a few of our favorite bars and had several drinks. She thought, as I did, that it was unjust to withhold money from us, yet give it to Craig.

On the way home from the bar, we stopped by the liquor store and stocked up on beer and wine. When I knew I would be drinking beer the rest of the day, and if I was out driving, I would stop at a liquor store on the way home, but save the store a block from my apartment for later — for when

I was drunk and couldn't drive — then I could just walk over there. I didn't want to have to visit the same liquor store twice in one day — except in a pinch.

I downed the six-pack, then walked back to the local liquor store and bought another one. By six o'clock I'd already had ten beers and not eaten very much, so I was pretty drunk. As I did often when I was drunk, I got my little address book out and started calling people I hadn't talked to in a long time. I never even wondered whether people could hear in my voice I was drunk, though I'm sure they knew.

After I'd called a few old friends, I called my dad. His wife Letitia answered and I shared my thoughts on how it wasn't fair that I didn't get the money because my brother had died in a car accident.

My dad got on the other line and held his ground. I went to an extreme. I said I was going to kill myself that night and that I didn't want to live anymore. I didn't especially want to die. I wanted to hurt my dad for keeping my money.

They both got upset. Letitia started crying hysterically. And then I even heard my dad cry. Before that, the only time I'd ever known of my dad crying was when my brother had died. I was stunned.

When he pulled himself together, he spoke to me firmly. "Linda, if you kill yourself tonight, I'll be upset for a week or two," he said. "But I'll get over it."

This wasn't working at all. I needed more leverage.

"I have to go now," I said flatly and hung up on them.

I wanted to be dramatic and make them wonder if I was out there killing myself. Thinking I was incredibly clever, I picked up the phone immediately to call someone else. I had to dial with one eye closed, so I could focus on the dialer. I had to make sure the line was busy if Dad and Letitia tried to call back.

After several minutes of talking to anyone who would talk to me, I started feeling like I might get sick. Everything was starting to spin. I hung up the phone and lay down.

When my dad finally did get through on the phone, Julie answered. He told her about our conversation and Julie came in to my room. She saw me lying face down on the bed.

"Well, she's not going to kill herself tonight, Dad," Julie told him. "She's passed out."

17

Behind Bars

Julie and I used to frequent a place called Rocky Galenti's. It was a party bar with music so loud — day or night — that you could never hear anyone talking, even if they were shouting. Luckily, the bartender knew what we wanted. As soon as she saw us come in, she'd start pouring a lite beer for me and a glass of wine for Julie.

There was something so comforting about being a regular. When I was at Rocky Galenti's, I stayed as long as I could. Usually, I'd go in around two in the afternoon and stay till nine or ten, when I started getting sleepy, and then I'd take a taxi home. During the course of the night, the bartender would give me a free drink or two and I got drunk nearly every time I went. I thought of Rocky Galenti's as a "happening" place.

Another regular once told me that she used to see me there, making the rounds, stopping at every seat to say something friendly to everybody. There must've been twenty-five seats at the bar and another one hundred people in the room, but that never stopped me.

That's how they knew me at Rocky Galenti's — outgoing and friendly. They never saw how that all changed when I went home.

* * *

On one occasion, I left the bar after several hours of

drinking and went to Steve's house. I didn't know it, but this was going to turn out to be one of the worse nights I ever had when I was drinking.

We started arguing as soon as he opened the front door. He could see at a glance I was drunk. He'd come to know the signs all too well. So he launched into his familiar attack: "Why are you here? You know I don't want to see you when you're like this. What's your problem? You're just using me. Why am I even with you, anyway? You're a drunk. What kind of a relationship is this?"

It went on and on. So boring. I could've run through his lines if he wasn't even there. I was yelling back, too, but I was saying all the things I'd said before. We'd been through this same fight so many times, I felt like I was watching myself in an endless re-run. There was no variation we hadn't tried before.

We seemed to be in some sort of drunken nightmare, yelling and screaming at each other, trying to get out, but we were trapped. Was that my fault? I'd just come over, looking for a little companionship. There was only one way out.

"I'm going to kill you!" I shouted.

I didn't really want to kill him, of course. I just wanted to scare him half to death. The adrenaline was pulsing inside me so hard that I had to do something "loud" to calm down.

I picked up a heavy ceramic ashtray from the coffee table. The thing probably weighed at least five pounds. Steve was facing the other way. "I swear to god," I screamed, rushing toward him. "I'm going to KILL you!"

Steve turned around to face me, lifting his fists up quickly to protect his face. His left hand slammed into my eye…

It really hurt!

I'd been in a rage, just moments before, but now all I could think about was my poor eye! I dropped the ashtray to the floor and it shattered into little pieces. I bawled like a baby.

"Oh, baby…" Steve said, coming toward me.

A loud pounding on the front door cut his sympathy short. "OPEN UP! POLICE!" Apparently a neighbor had called 911 to report the sound of a fight with someone screaming: "I'm going to kill you!"

When Steve let them in, I was in the bedroom, sitting on the bed, holding my eye and whimpering. One of the officers kneeled down in front of me and asked me to move my hands aside, so he could get a good look at it. "You're getting a black eye," he said. "You need to put some ice on it immediately to reduce the swelling. How did this happen?"

"Steve hit me," I shouted, bursting with self-pity.

"No, I didn't," Steve said, disgusted. "I was protecting myself. She was coming at me, holding that big ashtray and saying she was going to kill me. I just put my hand up and she ran into it."

"She ran into your hand?" the officer said, skeptically. "That's right," Steve insisted, getting angry. "Tell him, Linda."

After seeing the alarm on the officer's face, when he looked at my eye, I'd gone to the bathroom mirror to investigate. The skin below my eye was puffy and already starting to turn different colors. I was going to have a black eye — for the first time in my life.

There was still so much alcohol in my system that this felt like a complete tragedy to me, the saddest thing I'd ever heard. I started crying even harder.

"Listen, Miss, you can press charges, if you'd like," the officer said, standing at the bathroom door.

I liked the idea of that. My eye looked awful and it was all his fault.

But if I pressed charges, they'd take Steve away in handcuffs and the whole point — the thing that had brought me over here in the first place — was that I didn't want to be alone. I didn't want much. Why was it this hard to get what I wanted? Life was so unfair.

I ran some cold water on a washcloth, then came out of

the bathroom, holding it up to my eye. The cool cloth felt nice.

I looked at Steve and then the officers. "No. No charges," I said.

* * *

The next day, I woke up with my head pounding. I was so afraid to look in the mirror, but it had to be done. Crawling out of bed, I made my way to the bathroom. Might as well get it over with. For a brief moment, I thought it might be possible that the whole thing had been a dream and my face would look like nothing had happened. It felt right, but when I turned on the light and stared at my face in the mirror, there was a big, black shiner looking back at me. It was worse than I thought. Make-up was definitely not going to cover this. What was I going to say when people asked me, "What happened to you?"

"I don't even know how long a black eye lasts…" I muttered to myself. "A day? A week?"

Steve heard me mumbling in the bathroom and came to the doorway. He said to me, very sweetly, "Come here. Let me see what I did to you." When I turned around, he was startled by how big and black my eye was. "Ohmigod," he said and starting laughing.

"It's not funny," I whimpered, giving him a look that said I knew he was to blame.

"You do know I didn't hit you, right? You ran into me when I put my hand out."

"That's your story," I snapped. "You punched me. You never hit me before. I'll never forgive you." Whether he'd meant to hit me or not, I was going to have to go out with a big, black eye because of him. I wanted to make him nervous.

"Linda," he said. "You know that's not true."

"I'm going out," I said, putting on my darkest sunglasses. I had plans to meet Elizabeth for lunch.

Since I wasn't working, I was far too restless not to go

out and socialize during the day. During the day, the sunglasses would keep me from having to explain. When I went to coffee or lunch with someone, it was imperative that we sit outside, so I could keep my sunglasses on. If I wanted to go out after dark, I'd have to come up with a story. "I ran into Steve's hand when I was pretending to kill him when I was drunk" wouldn't work. I was going to need to come up with a more plausible lie.

They say the best lies have a convincing bit of truth mixed in. So I decided to build my lie around not one true thing, but two. Everyone who knew me well knew two things about me: I got drunk a lot and I slept with the fan on every night to keep from getting sick and to drown out the noise on the street. So my story was that I got drunk and tripped over the fan. It was perfect. I was sure it would work. And I think everyone I told that story to believed me. Except Elizabeth.

When we met at the coffee shop for lunch, I was wearing my sunglasses. We found a table and started chatting right away. With a close friend, like Elizabeth, it was going to be awkward to leave the glasses on the whole time, even at a sunny table. I'd have to take them off. But before I did, I tried out my perfect lie on Elizabeth.

"I don't get it," she said, frowning. "You tripped over the fan, but… how did your eye hit the fan?"

"What do you mean?" I asked, innocently.

"Well, I'm trying to picture it…" she persisted. "If you trip and the fan falls over, you're going to fall past it, right? I mean, your face wouldn't circle back around and hit the fan…"

"Look, I don't know, Elizabeth," I said, with an irritated tone, hoping to make her feel unreasonable for asking. "I was drunk, okay? I don't remember the details."

No one can really argue with that.

It took awhile for the black eye to go away, but, with Steve at least, I milked it for all it was worth. He couldn't help but feel a little guilty when he looked at me. So he went out of his way to be nice to me for the rest of that week. Until I pushed things too far.

* * *

Not wanting to sit at the bar where Steve worked, explaining my black eye to every new drunk who made a smart remark, I had decided to stay home. There was nothing to do but sit on the couch, watching soaps and drinking. Steve was working late and I'd called him several times on the job, as I got drunker and drunker.

"What time do you get off work?" I demanded, when I called around nine o'clock.

"You just asked me that thirty minutes ago, Linda," Steve said in a hostile tone. If he couldn't be happy at work, he should get another job! "I told you. Ten."

"Great. I'll come over…"

"No. Don't come over. I told you. You've been drinking since noon. You won't even be able to stand up by ten o'clock. Just stay home."

"Shut up! I can stand," I assured him.

At eleven I took a taxi from my apartment to Steve's place and knocked on the door. "Hey. It's me."

"Go away."

"Open the door."

"I said, go away. I don't want you here." Steve called, without opening the door.

We shouted back and forth for a few minutes, till he stopped talking and walked away from the door. Did he think he could ignore me? How ridiculous. From the porch, I could see that his side window was open. I walked over and popped out the screen.

"Oh, Steve?" I called. "If you don't let me in, I'll crawl through the window. It's not a problem. Really. Make your girlfriend crawl through the damn window in the middle of the night. Why not? You've already given me a BLACK EYE."

Steve opened the door. "Shh. Be quiet, for god's sake. Everyone in the neighborhood can hear you."

When I saw the door opened, I ran toward him and pushed my way into the house before he could close it again. As soon as we were inside, I was livid. I was yelling, screaming, creating a lot of drama. Steve kept begging me to calm down and go home.

"Just try to make me," I screamed.

"The police are on their way," he threatened.

"You're lying."

"No, I'm not. I called them before I let you in."

I couldn't tell if he was telling the truth or not. But I didn't want to see the police, if they came, so I grabbed a cigarette and went around to the side of the house to smoke. It was dark on that side. I moved up near the corner, where I could see the police car, if it pulled up, but the police wouldn't be able to see me. I took a long drag on my cigarette and leaned against the wall of the house. The streetlight was casting a long glow of light across the lawn in my direction, but it didn't reach me. I felt invisible, standing there. My eyes wanted to close. I was so drunk and tired.

What was taking them so long? Every minute felt like ten. He was bluffing. He'd never call the police. What a load of crap. I should just go back in and lie down. All I wanted to do now was sleep.

Then I saw lights slowly move into the driveway. I snapped awake and stepped back further around the corner, so I wouldn't be seen. When I peeked back around, there was another set of headlights. Two squad cars were parked in front of the house like tanks, blocking the escape of the enemy forces. It seemed like overkill for one noisy girlfriend.

The officers got out and knocked on Steve's door. I assumed he would send them away, telling them everything was under control. I was quieter now. That was what he wanted, right? I could hear their voices, but I couldn't make out what they were saying. Why were they talking so long? What was he telling them, his life story? I shouldn't have to stand around waiting like this. No woman should. God, I needed a new life... and a bathroom.

Desperately needing to go, I abandoned my hiding place and walked around the front of the house to the front door. I strolled right past the police officers talking to Steve, went into Steve's studio and locked the door.

While I was in the bathroom, I could hear a commotion outside, but I ignored it. When I finally came back out, I could hear it was Steve, knocking on the door, "Linda, come on! Open the door. The policemen want to talk to you."

"NO," I shouted. "Go away. I don't want you here."

After another ten or fifteen minutes of pleading, Steve finally persuaded me to open the door. "I'll pay for a cab to take you home," he said, as he came in.

"No. I'm staying here."

"Linda," he said, his voice cracking with anger. "You've got to go home."

I stepped toward him, angrily. "You can't make me go. I won't leave. I live here too."

"You've got to go. You do NOT live here. You have your own apartment."

"Shut up." I took a swing at him and hit him on his chest twice, hard. One of the officers stepped toward me. I spun around and hit the officer on the shoulder. He grabbed my arm before I could pull it back, twisted me around quickly and started putting me in handcuffs.

"That's it," the officer said, clearly out of patience. "You're going to county jail."

"NO," I screamed as loud as I could. He had me by one wrist, but I tried to wrangle around and keep my other hand free so he couldn't get the cuffs on. For a second I thought I could slip loose, but I guess he'd run into this kind of thing before. He grabbed my free hand and slapped the cuffs on before I knew what was happening.

"These are too tight. Let me go," I screamed, trying to

kick the policeman. The cuffs were actually so tight that they injured my left wrist. It hurt for years after that.

But in that moment, I didn't care about anything anymore. I couldn't stand being drunk and in handcuffs. It filled me with panic, as if I had a phobia about it. I HAD to get free somehow.

As the policeman dragged me out to the car and guided me into the back seat, Steve came after us, looking very distraught. I shouted accusations at him, trying to make him suffer. "This is all your fault. I don't want to see you anymore. I hate you."

When the policeman slammed the door, I broke down and cried.

* * *

It was strange to be in handcuffs in the back of a police car, behind the cage that divides the criminals from the cops. I'd been sure I could outsmart the cops, but here I was, locked in and headed for jail.

With few options left to me, I stopped crying and gave the policeman hell the whole way. As we neared the station, I started swearing at him at the top of my lungs. He stopped the car, turned around and swore right back at me, using exactly the same words. I was shocked. Cops aren't supposed to do that.

I threatened to sue him for police brutality. He told me to shut the f--- up.

"And I'm going to sue you for telling me to shut up and swearing at me," I muttered, sitting in my cage. I slumped down in the seat, pouting and sullen. I would've folded my arms across my chest, but they were chained behind my back.

When he finally brought me into the jail and booked me, I got to make my one phone call. I tried to call my dad collect, but I couldn't remember his phone number. I'd never had a problem remembering his number when I was sober. I came up with something that sounded right and asked the operator to give it a try.

It was well after midnight. A groggy man picked up the phone, fumbled with the receiver, then said hello. The operator told him he had a collect call from his daughter in lock-up at the county jail. Would he accept the charges?

"I don't have a daughter," the man said gruffly.

"I'm sorry, sir, I know we've woken you, but your daughter's in jail..." the operator insisted.

"That's not my dad," I told her.

"I don't have a daughter," he repeated.

We called my mom instead. I told her Steve had sent me to jail, then I burst into tears and hung up. Mom woke up her husband, then called Julie, and all three of them headed for the jail to bail me out.

* * *

When I was finally put into my cell, the reality hit me: I was in jail, and I couldn't leave. For the first time in my life, my freedom had been taken away from me.

I swore that I would make the jail personnel miserable all night for putting me in jail. For hours, I screamed as loud as I could, nonstop. They ignored me, but I knew I was pissing them off. Every so often, I screamed, "Help!" desperately, so someone would have to come and see if everything was all right.

My wrist still hurt from the handcuffs and I was cold in the cell. There was a small cot in the cell with a blanket the size of a baby blanket. When I stretched out on the cot, the blanket covered maybe half my body.

When one of the officers came by to check on me, I complained that I was cold and cried as pathetically as I could, but he gave me a hostile look. He must've known I'd been raising hell since they put me in the police car. The guy who arrested me was probably his best friend. I got the feeling he would've taken my half-blanket away from me, if he thought he'd get away with it.

As soon as I realized he wasn't going to help me, I started screaming and cussing at him until he left. Then I finally fell asleep on the little cot and slept for a few hours.

Meanwhile, my family had arrived to bail me out, but I was at war with the jail personnel and they weren't inclined to let me go. They said I had been making such a commotion that they were going to keep me in jail until morning. My mom would have to come back to pick me up.

Mom was alone when she picked me up the next morning. The sun was just coming up. It was a beautiful day. I remembering thinking that most people were getting ready for work and feeling great. Me, I was hung over. I didn't know whether I had a boyfriend or not. And I was just being released, after a long, cold night in jail.

Instead of thinking I could change my life and become one of those people who were getting ready for work and feeling great about their lives, I felt sorry for myself. I wanted to go back home, call Steve and get things back to the way they were. I didn't even consider that there might be a better way.

It was less than two months before I found myself back in jail again.

* * *

On another sunny afternoon in spring, I called a taxi and went bar hopping alone. I started off at a few of the bars where I knew people, but nothing much was happening and I was getting bored, so I decided to hit a few gay bars in town. I'd always gotten along with gay people, so I wasn't afraid of getting hit on by a woman.

I started at a gay bar Steve and I went to sometimes. Some of his friends were singers at this bar, so we would often stop by, even though we were one of the few straight couples there.

Just as the bartender brought me my lite beer, a flamboyant young guy, about twenty-five, sat down next to me. He introduced himself as Terry and started up a lively conversation. I had been drinking for a few hours by this time and before long, I found myself trying to talk him out of being gay. My argument was simple: It's just a bad idea to be gay.

"In my opinion," I told him, "Your life would be so much easier if you were straight."

Terry had had a few beers himself and seemed captivated by what I was saying. I was starting to think I may be changing a gay man to a straight man with all my straight talk. "Do you think a gay man could turn straight?" Terry asked.

"Oh, yeah. And with God, Terry, anything is possible. Remember that," I said, as I took another drag off my cigarette and gulped my beer.

I ordered another beer. By this time, the bar owner, a bald, stocky man with tattoos all over his body, had taken over behind the bar. Apparently, he'd been listening to my conversation with Terry. "I'm warning you," he told me, quietly. "You'd better watch it." He was obviously unhappy about something. I didn't see what that had to do with me. This guy needed to loosen up, have a beer … Terry and I were having a good time.

"Anyway," I said, sitting back down next to Terry. "I'm just saying, the world is such a difficult place. Why give yourself the added grief of being gay? People will pick on you — especially somebody as swishy and flamboyant as you are. I mean anybody could glance at you and know you were gay. So I'll bet you're constantly running into people who disapprove of your lifestyle, aren't you? No matter where you go, they're making fun of you, saying you're a sissy, calling you a faggot …"

"GET THE HELL OUT OF MY BAR." Suddenly, the

Grim One was standing next to us. He pointed toward the door.

"Can I at least finish my beer?" I whined.

"NO. LEAVE NOW OR I'LL CALL THE COPS."

"You'd better go," Terry said, apologizing with his voice. "He owns the bar. He'll do it."

Stubborn as ever, I stayed a few more minutes to see if he'd make me leave. I guzzled the rest of my beer. Well, I paid for it. Then I walked outside and stood by the front door, smoking a cigarette.

Terry had said he'd call a taxi for me. Apparently, the owner had a better idea. Within a few minutes, a police car pulled up. Two policemen got out in front of the bar and stood next to me.

"You were asked to leave the premises," the first one said. "You need to get completely away from the bar."

"Will you take me home?" I asked, thinking they could save me money for a taxi.

"No," the other one said. "We'll call you a taxi."

Nothing was going my way. First the bar owner, now these guys. What the hell was the problem? I got argumentative. "I can't take a taxi. I don't have any money. Are you going to take me home or not?"

"Just leave then, or we'll have to take you to jail."

"Ohhh," I said. "Jail? Now I'm really scared. Is that all you've… " In mid-sentence, my legs suddenly gave out and I fell to the ground.

I heard one of the officers say, "Throw her in the car. Let's go."

The policemen picked me up off the ground and flopped me down in the back of the police car. I spent another night in jail. But I wasn't alone this time. I shared a cell with three other women. One of them was a waitress who had worked with Julie.

This time, I didn't call my mom. And I didn't bother to give anyone at jail a problem, because I knew the drill. I thought maybe, if I was a nice prisoner, I might get out that night, but we were all released back into the sunshine the next morning.

* * *

My fourth run-in with the police happened again at Steve's house. I have no recollection of that episode at all.

What I do remember is going to court. I was assigned a public defender and I lied to him. "You have to get the judge to understand," I said, as earnestly as I could. "That experience in jail really changed me. I haven't had a drink since I got out."

The public defender dutifully wrote that down. It looked so true and official on his yellow legal pad that it inspired me to embellish things a bit.

"And…" I smiled, "I've started going to church again."

He looked up, innocently.

"Every week. I will never live that kind of life again, thank the Lord. I've changed."

When I stood before the judge, I put on my most winning smile and repeated the same spiel. With the public defender nodding beside me and confirming everything in his notes, the judge granted me two years' probation. He also said he'd like me to attend twenty AA meetings. "You don't have to verify for this court that you've attended those meetings. With your new attitude about giving up alcohol for good, I trust that you'll want to go — for your own good."

"Thank you, Your Honor," I said gratefully. I shook the public defender's hand, then left immediately to meet Julie at the Four Winds. We both got drunk that night.

18

The Wedding Incident

BEFORE I MET STEVE, I WAS DATING A GUY NAMED BOB. Denise, who had been my friend since junior high school, was dating Chip. Chip and Bob got along marvelously. All four of us went out for drinks and dinner together several times. I always drank too much, of course, but Chip liked to drink a lot too. Usually, Denise and Bob would stay fairly quiet and drink very little, while Chip and I became the life of the party. Chip was loud and animated — and hysterically funny — when he was buzzed. We always had a great time.

After about a year, Denise and Chip decided to get married. By that time, I was dating Steve. Denise told me her good news one night when she and I were having dinner alone. I said I was excited they were getting married, even though I was jealous of her happiness.

"I'd like you to be my maid of honor," she smiled.

I smiled too, trying to look happy and honored that she had picked me to be her maid of honor. And I agreed, of course. But my heart wasn't in it.

Even though we'd grown up with each other and she was a dear friend, I told myself, for some reason, that we weren't that close. I took it for granted that Denise was my friend and would always be my friend, but I'd always thought of Elizabeth as my best friend. When Denise asked me to be her maid of honor, I thought it was because she didn't have any other close friends.

All I could think about was how much work it would be

for me. So when Denise's older sister Mary started doing all the work the maid of honor is supposed to do, I welcomed it. Mary was one of the bridesmaids, but she never asked me to do anything except go to the bridal shower, rehearsal and the wedding itself. I was relieved.

Before the rehearsal, I'd had about four beers to drink and things had not gone all that well. I can't say exactly what went wrong, but I didn't quite seem to be doing everything the way I was supposed to. Denise's mom looked irritated with me. She'd always been crazy about me in the past, but at the dinner after the rehearsal, she seemed distant and displeased, as if I'd done something wrong. As usual, I just had another drink and tried not to think about it.

The wedding itself went well. It was held at the Lady of Mount Carmel, a small, but elegant, Mediterranean-style church in Montecito — the wealthiest neighborhood in Santa Barbara, which is already one of the most expensive cities in the world. The ceremony was lovely and all the guests seemed happy for Denise and Chip. Personally, I was looking forward to the reception, because I knew there would be an open bar.

Steve was going to be meeting me at the reception around two o'clock. I'd asked him not to come to the wedding because I was afraid I'd be nervous if I knew he was watching me, and I'd make a mistake.

While I waited for him to show up, I had a glass of wine. It was such a formal setting. I was wearing heels and lavender chiffon. Wine just seemed more ladylike.

"I miss drinking wine," I told myself, as I took another graceful sip. Wine didn't bloat me like beer did. And it gave me a nice glow, too.

By three o'clock, Steve hadn't arrived. Since he worked just a few miles away, I couldn't imagine what was keeping him. I danced with a few of the guests and socialized while I drank one glass of wine after another.

An hour or so later, I was really starting to feel

annoyed. Where was my date? I hadn't even asked that he attend the wedding. (Guys always hate that anyway.) Now he couldn't even make it to the reception?

Muttering under my breath, I stepped outside to have a cigarette, just as Steve pulled up in front of the reception hall in a car I had never seen before.

"You're two hours late, you know." I said, snapping at Steve, more like a fishwife than a lady in lavender chiffon.

"My car broke down. Some guy at the bar let me use his car for a few hours."

"The reception is practically over. I told you that car would give you trouble. Why didn't you listen to me? I can't even depend on you to do a simple thing like show up to a reception."

"You can't depend on me?" Steve said, ready for a fight.

After the frustration of having his car break down, he was in no mood to be attacked. Within a few minutes he was threatening to leave.

"Leave?" I snapped. "No. Don't you dare leave me. I need a ride home."

"Where's your car?"

"I can't drive. I've been drinking," I said sternly, turning my back on him and walking back toward the reception. Halfway up the stairs, I stepped on my dress and almost fell, but somehow managed to keep my balance. I thought Steve would be there to take my arm, but he was still fuming, leaning against that stranger's car.

I could see what was going on in his head. "Don't leave," I warned him, pointing my finger at him, to let him know I meant it.

When I got back inside, I quickly accepted another glass of wine. The glasses were small, but it was probably my sixth glass. In no time at all, I was feeling on top of the world. The wine was good and everyone looked so lovely. I started swaying to the music. When a slow song came on, I made my way over to Chip.

"Chip, I would like to dance with the groom, if I may," I said in my most ladylike manner. Chip was tall and I loved dancing with tall men. I didn't realize that no one but the bride should dance a slow dance with the groom.

"Not now," Chip said. "Maybe the next song."

I thought he was just playing hard to get, so I just pulled his arm and tugged him out onto the dance floor. When she saw what was happening, Denise smiled at me. Until that night, I could do no wrong in Denise's eyes. Chip resisted at first and then he laughed and gave in.

We were the only ones on the dance floor. The music was sultry and romantic. As high as I was, I abandoned myself to the music, closing my eyes and feeling into the mood. I forgot I was dancing with Chip and started dancing way too close, pressing my hips into him and rubbing my entire body against him, hard. The whole room must have been watching us. The tension must have been rising, but I didn't even feel it. In my imagination, I was having a romantic, private dance with Steve. My lips were at his ear. I slid my face down further and placed a big, wet kiss on his neck.

"I have to go dance with my bride," Chip said harshly. He pulled away from me and stalked back across the room to be with Denise.

It was so startling that it snapped me out of my haze. I stood alone for a moment on the dance floor, staring after him in horror. What had I done?

Denise never spoke to me again.

* * *

Eventually, Steve had had about all he could take.

So much for my brilliant plan to date a bartender so I could keep drinking.

If he had been any other guy, I would've blown it off. I'd done it many, many times before. As soon as a guy started giving me a hard time, trying to tell me when to drink, I was gone. It was over.

The trouble was, I loved Steve. So when Steve said that if I stopped drinking, it would be "the best present I could ever give him," no matter how much I wanted not to care, I did care, just a little.

I knew I wouldn't quit drinking forever. I didn't want to. But I did quit drinking — for Steve — for eighty-nine days.

It was like a game to me to see how long I could go without a beer, but I never considered quitting for good. It was just a present. Though I didn't mention that to Steve. When he saw I was sticking to it, he got his hopes up. He started believing that I really might quit drinking for good. It made him happy and I was glad for that, while it lasted. But after eighty-nine days, I'd had enough.

On the ninetieth day, Steve was getting dressed for a funeral. His grandfather had died earlier in the week. After the funeral, the family was going to meet for dinner at his father's house, so he'd be gone for several hours.

Steve had been close to his grandfather. It was an upsetting time for him, but he was coping with it fairly well. He dug out the family photo albums to search for any photos of his grandfather he could find. There they were at a cabin together, when Steve was five. It must've been a family vacation. Steve couldn't remember anything about it, except for something about chasing a chipmunk throwing pine needles one afternoon. But in the photo, his grandfather had an arm around him and he looked so proud. Steve stared at the photos for hours, trying to stir up bits of memories to hold onto now that his grandfather was gone. I listened to the stories and felt sorry that there was so little I could do.

We'd been spending a lot of quality time together during my eighty-nine days of sobriety. We'd grown a lot closer and had had a lot of fun. Steve certainly seemed much happier. And I hadn't missed drinking as much as I'd thought I would.

But if he was going to be gone for hours, and he'd be drinking I wanted to drink too. I wasn't invited to go to the funeral. What I really wanted was simple. I just wanted to go to a bar and have a beer.

Steve came over and kissed me before he left. He told me how proud he was of me for going so long without drinking and smiled at me with affection. I loved it when he looked at me like that.

"So, what are you going to do today?" he said, picking up his car keys, as he headed toward the door.

"Julie and I are going out for a few drinks," I said, casually.

Steve froze. "Bottled water?" he said, but his eyes were wide with alarm. He knew exactly what I meant.

Bottled water. That was another reason to start drinking again! For eighty-nine days, whenever I went out to a bar, I'd always gotten bottled water — I hated bottled water. Other people were drinking booze and I was drinking Perrier or Crystal Geyser. I was paying for water.

Steve hadn't moved. "You aren't going to drink are you?" he said stiffly.

"Just a few beers."

His face changed completely. He looked so disappointed with me, but that didn't change my mind. I'd always known it would only be a matter of time before I'd drink again and today was the day. The ninetieth day. Why not? I'd proven to myself that I could stop for almost three months. If I could do that, then I didn't have as much of a problem as I'd thought — or as everybody had thought.

If I had a problem with alcohol, could I have stopped for eighty-nine days? Of course not. There was no problem. I might as well end this marathon now. Then at least, I — and everybody else — could stop with the counting down the days, wondering, "When is Linda going to drink again?"

When he started talking, Steve sounded like he was

going to cry. "I'm going to my grandfather's funeral," he said softly, trying to retain his composure. "I loved my grandfather and I love you. I'm asking you … Linda … please don't drink today. Okay?"

Our eyes met, but I didn't say anything. How could I? He didn't want to hear what I wanted to say.

"Do it for me. Please. Will you promise that?" Steve said. "Just today. This is a difficult day for me …" He could tell from the look on my face that the answer was no. Something shifted in his eyes. The pain stepped back, behind a shield. "If you do drink, don't be here when I get home."

"Okay," I said, and kissed him as he shut the door.

* * *

Julie wasn't surprised when I called. I think she'd been biding her time until I started drinking again — counting the days, like everybody else.

"It's happy hour!" I said, when she picked up the phone. Julie just laughed.

Julie and I went out for a few drinks. I got high quickly from the beer since I hadn't had a drink in so long. Not wanting to worry about driving while buzzed, I picked up a six-pack of Miller Lite after Julie and I decided to leave the bar, and drank them all before Steve got home.

When he came in, he stood in the middle of the living room and stared hard at me. "Are you drunk?"

I thought I'd distract him. I got up off the couch and walked toward him, with my arms outstretched to hug him. "No, of course not," I said, giving him a big smile. I was very buzzed for two reasons: I hadn't had a drink in eighty-nine days and then I'd had eight beers in six hours. I might've been swaying a bit.

"You are drunk."

"I'm not! I only had three beers. I'm just not used to it."

I laughed, knowing that this was a funny thing for me to be saying.

Steve wasn't laughing. "All I asked was for you not to drink on the day of the funeral and you couldn't do that. I can't trust you, can I?"

Ordinarily, I would've felt bad. I knew he loved his grandfather. And I knew how much it meant to him for me to quit drinking — not just on the day of the funeral, but any day of the week. It was true that our relationship had been so much better those eighty-nine days. But I wasn't thinking about any of that. I was disappointed with Steve for telling me he couldn't trust me to not drink.

19

Cat Fight

WHEN I DRANK I HATED SILENCE. THERE WAS NOTHING AS terrifying as being alone with my own thoughts.

So many of the things going on in my life were difficult to even think about. Whenever a quiet moment snuck up on me, I tormented myself with incidents that happened when I was drunk. Even if I managed to seem like I was blissfully unaware of them as they were happening, they caught up with me later. I'd be doing something innocuous — making the coffee or brushing my teeth — and the memory of some humiliating incident would flash before my mind. And I'd wince at the thought of it. I could see myself laughing it off or defending myself at the time. But without the buzz of alcohol in my veins, nothing seemed quite as amusing or defensible.

Some mornings, I'd get up and lean on the bathroom sink, in front of the mirror, afraid to even turn on the light and see my face. I was living hard, filling my body with toxins, smoking too much, eating too much, staying out too late and having the kind of experiences that really take a toll on your body, no matter what age you are.

More and more, the woman who stared back at me in the bathroom mirror looked ashen and dreadful. I had bags under my eyes and seemed thrashed. If I had a fight with Steve about my drinking the night before, it was even worse. Then I'd wake up, not only seriously hung over, but puffy-eyed from crying before bed. Most evenings, after a certain point, I didn't always remember what had happened, but my body remembered. I could see the remnants of the night on my face. There was no doubt about it. I was wearing myself out.

It was starting to wear on Steve too. Eventually, my drinking episodes started to make him cautious. If I cleaned up for a day — determined to have a great time with him, so he'd still want to hang around me — he didn't buy into it, as he had in the beginning. He'd be guarded and cynical. "This isn't real," he seemed to be telling himself. "It's just an act. She'll be right back to drinking and making our lives miserable tomorrow." And he'd hold back. Instead of joining in with me, he'd smile sadly and brush me off. Instead of getting excited about doing something I knew he loved, he'd hold back, letting me know that he had reservations and that he wasn't so willing to go along anymore.

He was also trying to punish me. It was as if he thought that if he pulled back and wasn't his usual self, I'd learn my lesson. I'd worry about losing him or feel bad about making him unhappy. Then I'd stop drinking so much.

It never worked.

I could see what he was doing, but it didn't make me feel bad or worry. I knew it was a game. And I was better at it than he was. I knew how to play him. So I'd turn the tables and make him feel guilty for being so distant and withdrawn.

I did love him, but I wasn't thinking about Steve in those moments. I was thinking about myself. The only thing on my mind was that I had no intention of being punished for doing what I wanted to do. If I wanted to drink, I was going to do it. And nothing Steve or anybody else could do would change me. I was not willing to accept any consequences for my actions whatsoever.

So until I stopped drinking, things just kept getting worse and worse.

* * *

One night, I was over at Steve's house drinking while he

was at work. His landlady, an older woman named Marla, had hinted that she didn't like it when I was there alone. "Linda spends an awful lot of time in the studio when you're not there," she'd said, the last time Steve paid the rent. She never came out and said I couldn't be there, but her tone of voice made it perfectly clear what she meant.

Steve had such a good deal on the rent that he didn't want to blow it. So he told me not to come over when he wasn't home. But he didn't ask for my key.

So there I was, with my six-pack, curled up on his couch watching television, when I heard Marla screaming at the top of her lungs.

Steve's studio was connected to the main house, where Marla lived with her boyfriend, Ted. They fought with each other all the time when they were drunk. Or at least we assumed they were fighting. All we could ever hear was Marla, screaming and yelling at Ted. If Ted said anything back, you couldn't hear it through the wall.

Once or twice, I'd tiptoe over and lean my ear against the wall to see if I could hear anything come out of his mouth. "Come on, Ted!" I'd mumble, rooting for him. "Are you going to sit there and take that? Let her have it!" But he never did.

This time, I was too drunk to get involved. I just moaned and rolled my eyes, then turned up the volume on the TV.

A few minutes later Steve came home. The door opened just as I was lifting a beer to my mouth. Leaning against the couch on the floor were the last two cans of Miller Lite, still clinging to the plastic rings of the six-pack. It was clear from the glaze in my eyes where the other cans had gone.

As Steve opened his mouth to say something, there was a sudden crash from the main house. It sounded like Marla had fallen over or had started hurling furniture at Ted. I could easily picture her picking up the coffee table and throwing it at him. Before he could say a word to me, Steve turned and ran next door to see if everything was all right.

It got quiet over there for awhile. I chugged down the rest of my beer and started wondering what was going on. Had she hit him with the table? Were they both lying dead on the floor? Feeling gutsy, I meandered over there to see for myself.

When I got there, Marla was standing just inside the living room, talking to Steve with the front door open. Ted was nowhere in sight. As soon as she saw me, Marla started shouting and carrying on. She was so drunk that her words slurred together. "Hey, Steve! I thought I told you Linda can't be here when you're not home!" She waved her can of beer in my direction and scowled at me.

"Marla, I AM home," Steve said, as if that settled it. He put his arm around me and patted my shoulder. It looked like he was ready to go home. But this was a fight I'd been waiting for.

I walked through the door into Marla's living room and said, "That is SO UNFAIR. Steve pays the rent. He can do whatever he wants in his own place. I can be here if he wants me to be here — whether he's home or not."

Marla was more than ready for a fight too. "No, it's MY house. And I don't want you in my house when he's not here." She started coming toward me, swaying a bit and taking swipes at the air with her beer can. I thought she was going to hit me, so I put up my arm to protect my face. "Aw, look. I scared her." Marla howled. "I'm so scary. Ooo. Watch out." She practically doubled over with laughter, right next to me. So I pushed her — probably a little bit harder than I realized.

Marla staggered backward into her kitchen and caught herself on the counter. Then she glared up at me with true anger. Her eyes were so glossy from the alcohol that she really did look scary. She let out a yell and pushed herself off of the counter, lunging toward me. "GET OUT OF MY HOUSE," she screamed.

I turned to get out of her way, but her hand came up at me so fast. Before I knew it, she'd grabbed my hair and started pulling. I thought she'd rip my hair right out of my head. I screamed as loudly as I could, hoping she'd let go, but she didn't. So I grabbed her hair and started pulling. I hadn't been there for two minutes and we were in the middle of a full-blown cat fight.

Screaming and howling and pulling each other's hair, we fell down hard onto the kitchen floor and started rolling around. The alcohol in both our systems heated us up all the more. We were crying and yelling our guts out.

Steve stood over us, straddling our legs and trying to pull us apart, but we were locked together.

"Get out of my house," Marla kept repeating.

And I kept screaming back. "Let go of me. Let go."

We were both so drunk that we were stronger and more determined than Steve. He gave up and walked out of the room in disgust, cursing under his breath.

Finally, Marla yanked on my hair so hard that I started crying hysterically and she let go. As I struggled to get back up to my feet, Marla was still down on the linoleum, rolling around, sopping drunk. When she saw I was still within range, she gave me a little kick. I quite naturally kicked her back and we went at it again for a minute, kicking back and forth like second graders in a playground fight, calling each other every name we could think of. But I had had it. I just wanted to go home.

As soon as Steve stepped back into the kitchen, I pushed past him, shaking and crying. As I ran through the living room, I noticed Ted, sitting meekly in the corner with his head down, not even daring to get involved. I ran back down to our own couch and burst into tears. Steve was right behind me.

"Did you see that?" I sobbed. "Did you see poor Ted? He was like a little whipped puppy. She probably does this to him all the time. What a lunatic."

The woman had just attacked me. I expected Steve to sit down next to me, wrap his arms around me and console me. But he wasn't anywhere near me. He was skulking around the room, avoiding my eyes.

"That's just great," he muttered. "Now you've done it. She's definitely going to kick me out now. How could you do that to me, Linda? I can't believe it. You know how important this place is to me. I'll never find rent like this anywhere. Now I'll have to move… You're so selfish when you're drunk."

"It's not my fault. The woman attacked me," I cried.

Steve just glared at me. "Don't talk to me right now."

Steve went outside to be alone. I sat grimly on the couch and smoked a cigarette. My life was crap. There were no two ways about it. All I wanted was to have a few beers and watch TV till my boyfriend got home and now this. The woman attacks me and somehow… it's STILL my fault. Totally unfair.

The next morning, the fight with Marla was the first thing I thought of, before I opened my eyes. I lay there for a few minutes, thinking about the antics of the night before. Steve was like a son to Marla. She wasn't going to kick him out, I was sure. But I'd probably not be able to come around there again. I'd blown it for myself.

When he got up, Steve begged me to apologize to Marla. I told him I'd think about it, but Marla was the one who'd lunged at me. She was more at fault than I was. "She should apologize to me," I said. But Steve didn't see it that way and I knew Marla wouldn't either.

My solution was to stay away from Steve's house for a few days, while I thought things over. I felt embarrassed about the whole incident. The last thing I wanted to do was talk to Marla again. It was easy to imagine her holding it over me, gloating. I remembered her ridiculing me for putting my arm up to protect my face. That was something minor. What would she say about this?

I couldn't stand the thought of facing her, but before long, my desire to be at Steve's house was greater than my desire to avoid the situation so I picked up the phone and called Marla. The sooner I apologized, the sooner I could spend the night at Steve's.

To my surprise, Marla was very gracious. Most likely, she was just as embarrassed as I was. "We were both drunk and did some things that weren't nice," she said. "I'm sorry too. Maybe you and I could go out for coffee some time."

"Yes, I'd like that," I said, knowing we'd never go out for coffee.

Whenever I ran into her, after that, Marla always went out of her way to be courteous to me. I can't be sure she remembered much of our cat fight, but the memory of the two of us, pulling each other's hair out on the floor was hard for me to forget.

It was definitely one of the low points in my drinking days. I find it hard to believe that things could sink lower than that, but somehow they did.

20

Easter Fiasco

Two months before I stopped drinking, my mom and her husband Mel invited Julie and me over for dinner, the night before Easter.

I knew that Mom would only serve us one or two glasses of wine all night, so I prepared myself by drinking several beers before I went over there. I wanted to be sure to get enough alcohol into my system to make it through the night. Julie joined me for a few of those drinks.

Mel prepared a wonderful dinner of roast turkey and potatoes with sage and onions. He made my favorite corn salsa to go along with it. All during dinner, we enjoyed each other's company and had a lively conversation. There was classical music playing softly in the background and two candles burning on the table.

After my two allotted glasses of wine (on top of the beer), I was feeling buzzed and talkative. Before long, a giddy glow came over me. As I looked around at my family and the beautifully prepared dinner table, I was ecstatic. And I loved feeling that way. The only thing missing was someone to share it with — not just family, but a man. Preferably a man who would ply with me alcohol and have his way with me.

As usual on Saturday nights, Steve wasn't around. He made the most money on Saturdays, so he tried to work them if he could. But it left me alone on Saturday nights. And in this case, that was a mistake.

While Julie was telling Mom about a funny incident I'd

already heard, I excused myself from the table to go make a phone call to Nadir.

A few weeks before, I'd met Nadir at the office. I worked for an accountant at the time. Nadir was one of our wealthiest clients. He was an attractive Middle Eastern man, probably Iranian. When he'd come by on April 15 to meet with my boss Tom about his tax returns, there had been a little spark between us.

While Tom was looking over his file, Nadir kept glancing over at me. I smiled a little when our eyes met. After a few minutes, I excused myself, saying I was going outside for a cigarette. Nadir quickly joined me.

As I placed the cigarette between my lips, he offered me a light. I couldn't help but notice a certain chemistry, as he leaned in toward me. "You know, you live on the same street as my mom," I told him, letting the smoke escape slowly from my mouth.

"Really?" he said, watching me closely as he took a drag from his own. He reached in his pocket and pulled out his card. "If you're ever at your mother's house and you'd like to come by my place, give me a call," he smiled.

I shouldn't have taken the card since I'd been dating Steve for over two years. But I liked the thought that another man was interested in me, so I took it anyway, never thinking I'd call. At nine o'clock the night before Easter, when my boyfriend had left me alone and I was getting drunk, it suddenly seemed like a good idea. The family part of the evening was over, but the night was still young. And Nadir was just a block or two away…

A woman answered the phone when I rang. I immediately assumed Nadir either had a girlfriend or was married. I had nothing to lose, so I boldly asked to speak to Nadir anyway. What could she do, hang up on me?

Nadir came to the phone.

"I was going to stop by, but it sounds like you have company," I told him.

"No, that's my roommate," he said. "I have two female roommates. Are you at your mother's now?"

"Yes…" I said, suggestively.

"Why don't you come over?"

"Maybe I will. Do you have any wine?" I knew it was rude, but it was important to me. If he hadn't had any alcohol, I would've had to go get some. It's what a good guest would do anyway, so it wouldn't seem out of place.

"Of course. We have a lot of wine," Nadir assured me.

"I'll be there in a few minutes."

When I hung up the phone, I smiled. Now things were really starting to get exciting. I wasn't especially excited about seeing Nadir, but I wanted to spend the night drinking and I might as well do that at somebody's house. In that neighborhood, it was probably a beautiful house, too, which would only make the wine more enjoyable.

I'd decided to take a taxi home from Nadir's place when I was ready to go home. It meant I could drink with abandon and not have to worry about driving.

The only problem was that I couldn't let Mom know I was driving up the street to drink with some Iranian guy I barely knew. It wouldn't have gone over very well with her. So I was going to have to use a little ingenuity. Luckily, when I was starting to feel buzzed, I felt like the cleverest, most ingenious person in the world.

Feeling good about the way the night was progressing, I strolled back into the living room and visited with the family for a few minutes. As soon as I could catch Julie's eye, I gave her a look that let her know I wanted to leave. No one else would've recognized it, but Julie and I had worked out these looks since childhood. She knew exactly what I meant. Before long, Julie yawned and said she was starting to feel sleepy. I said I was too. Then we got up to leave.

It was handy that we'd come in separate cars that night. We often drove our own cars to Mom's house, even though we lived together. That way, one of us could leave early if we wanted to. Mom came outside to see us off. I drove down the street, as if I were following Julie home, then I quickly did a U-turn and drove back up the street toward Mom's house. I slowed as I approached, to make sure she'd gone back inside, then I cruised on past to Nadir's house, the very last house on the street.

It was too dark to see much of the landscaping or the house itself, but I could see that he had a view of the entire city.

When I knocked, Nadir opened the door and stepped outside to hug me. "It's so good to see you, Linda. Come in and meet my roommates."

Nadir's two roommates, Mara and Catrice, were attractive women around forty. They had long, straight hair, like hippies, and they were friendly and outgoing. By the time I arrived, they'd had dinner and a few glasses of wine as well. The four of us sat around for hours, drinking and talking. I can't remember a thing we talked about, because I had quickly crossed the line between buzzed and drunk.

Eventually, the two girls went to bed, leaving Nadir and me alone on the couch. He turned to kiss me and I leaned into him. Being drunk, I felt amorous toward Nadir. We enjoyed making out on the couch for awhile, until I had an odd sensation. I pulled away from Nadir and sat back on the couch.

"My head is spinning," I said, holding my palm against my forehead. "I think I need to lie down..." I stood up to walk to the bedroom and that's the last thing I remember.

On Easter morning, I woke up in Nadir's bed. He was lying next to me, sound asleep. I looked under the covers and discovered that I was still wearing my slip, but the dress I'd been wearing the night before was down on the floor next to my shoes. My underwear was bunched up at the foot of the bed.

What had happened? I tried to remember taking my clothes off or even coming into the bedroom, but I couldn't remember a thing.

"Well, if I can't remember anything, nothing probably

happened," I assumed, as I dragged myself out of bed.

I bent over to gather up my clothes and noticed I was still drunk. I needed some coffee soon or it was going to take a long time getting started this morning. I went into the bathroom to get dressed and rub some toothpaste on my teeth, so I could get rid of the ghastly taste of hangover breath.

When I came back to the bedroom, Nadir was awake, sitting up in bed smoking. "Good morning beautiful," he smiled, with a twinkle in his eyes.

Oh my God! Maybe I was wrong. That was not the look a man wore after nothing happened. I felt a kind of panic. I thought about Steve. He'd always told me if I ever slept with another man — even if I were drunk — our relationship would be over. Surely I hadn't slept with Nadir.

I stood in the bathroom doorway, staring at him, while he smiled and took another satisfied drag off his cigarette. Oh God. I was so afraid to ask him the question I needed to ask. My throat was dry. But I asked that awful morning-after question anyway in a monotone voice: "We didn't do anything last night, did we?"

"What do you mean?" he said, looking disappointed. "You wanted me. You came on to me."

"But did anything happen?" I asked again, more impatiently this time.

"Yes. You wanted to be with me," Nadir explained, getting out of bed and walking toward me.

"Stay away from me," I screamed. I don't know what came over me. All I could think was that the worst had happened — I'd finally done something that would cost me my relationship with Steve. I couldn't stand it. Suddenly, that Easter morning, I realized that none of the things I'd done when I was drunk — insulting people, getting kicked out of bars, getting arrested, losing friends — nothing would be as bad as losing Steve. It was too much to bear. I started crying and yelling at Nadir.

"Linda, what's wrong with you?" he said, alarmed.

"Don't cry. Please. Come here now," he said gently, reaching out for me.

"Get away from me." I screamed and burst into tears.

My scream woke Mara and Catrice. They knocked on the door, then came running into the room. "What's wrong?" they cried. "What happened?"

Nadir stood back from me, shaking his head. I could tell he wanted to comfort me, but he looked uncertain about what to do.

I didn't care. All I could think of was Steve. I had to tell him. I felt like I was already arguing with him, trying to defend myself. I had to try to make him see I hadn't meant it, try to get him to change his mind about leaving me. I had to get home.

I picked up my purse and started walking toward the door. Nadir blocked my way. "Look, Linda, I can't let you leave like this. Don't go." He grabbed my arm and I panicked.

"Let go of me. I'm calling the police," I screamed, trying to scare him, so he'd let go of me and I could leave. I picked up the phone on the table and dialed 911.

When Nadir saw what I was doing, his tone changed. He wasn't concerned about me now, he was angry. "Put the phone down, Linda," Nadir said sternly, trying to get closer.

I had dialed 911, but the receiver wasn't up to my ear. I hadn't realize the police were on the phone and could hear us.

"911..." the operator said in the background.

"Hello... this man raped me," I howled.

"Ahhh," Nadir cried.

"Tell the man the police are on the phone with you. Tell me the address and we'll send someone right over."

I told the police officer Nadir's address.

Nadir turned pale. The look he wore was as close to utter panic as I've ever seen on a man's face. He reached for the phone to explain himself to the officer.

"Stay back," I screamed, backing toward the wall, with the phone in my hand.

Nadir stepped back and looked at me in disbelief. What had happened to the party girl from the night before? he must've wondered. Mara and Catrice looked confused too.

Every time one of them got within ten feet of me, I'd hold my hand up and scream, "Stay back." The officer stayed with me on the phone for a few minutes more, while the three of them huddled together across the room from me, whispering to one another. I can only imagine what they must've been saying.

"The police are coming," I shouted at them, nearly hysterical.

By the time I'd made a few more calls, things had escalated beyond my control. First, I called Elizabeth to tell her I'd been raped, then I started crying all over again. Since it was Easter morning, she was with her mom, her husband and her two small children, celebrating. She said she was so sorry for what had happened and told me to call her later that day. "I'll be praying for you," she said.

Then I called Julie who was working overtime on Easter. She'd known I was going over to Nadir's house the night before, but she was horrified to hear what had happened. Every time I said, "I was raped," I started crying all over again. I needed some sympathy.

Mara and Nadir were in the living room talking when Catrice came back in and said, matter-of-factly, "The police are here."

I finished talking to Julie, then hung up the phone and walked outside. To my surprise, there were four police cars blocking the drive. It seemed like they'd sent an army to do the job of a single officer. I'd expected one policeman to show up. This was turning out to be a much bigger production than I'd thought it would be.

Nadir was already standing by one of the police cars in handcuffs. Mara was talking to two other policemen, while Catrice stood next to her, crying.

"You're just as guilty as Nadir," Catrice shouted, when

she saw me. "YOU came on to Nadir. I saw you." Mara just glowered at me and nodded her head. "I'll testify to that," she said, insisting he write it down.

The police officers glanced over at me, but their gaze was neutral, professional. After all they'd seen, they were probably willing to believe anything. One of them asked my name, address and phone number. While he was writing it down, I tried to remember coming onto Nadir. I couldn't remember it at all. Was Mara right? Had I come onto him? It was pretty painful to admit, standing there on the lawn with four police cars blocking the drive and Nadir being carted off to jail, but I didn't really doubt that I had come onto Nadir. It sounded exactly like something I'd do.

"Linda, tell them to let Nadir go," Mara pleaded. "You have the power to do that. Please."

"What are you doing? He's our friend," Catrice said harshly. "You know he didn't hurt you!"

"He raped me," I yelled at them. The more they tried to blame me for all this hassle, the surer I became of myself. I wished they'd just shut up and leave.

Maybe I had come on to Nadir. In fact, maybe I had come over to have a little fun and a few glasses of wine. He was an attractive guy. Maybe I was even hoping to have sex. But if you're blacked out and someone takes advantage of you, that's rape.

* * *

After the police took Nadir away in handcuffs, one of the officers said that if I were going to press charges, they would have to take me to the local hospital, so I could have a "rape exam." I got in the police car and cried all the way to the hospital.

It was a beautiful, sunny Easter morning. When I was a kid, Easter morning used to be so special. I'd get up and put on a beautiful pastel-colored dress, with little patent leather shoes and lacy white socks as I got ready for church. I always knew that sometime during the day, there was going to be an Easter egg hunt and a chocolate candy bunny.

But not this Easter. This year I was sitting in the back of a police car, going to get a rape exam.

I felt dirty and just wanted to take a shower, but it would be hours before I could do that. My head was pounding from the hangover. The whole morning was starting to feel surreal.

When we arrived, I checked into the hospital and a nurse took me to my room. The police officer waited outside the door. The nurse instructed me to take off my clothes and put them in a bag. Then she gave the bag to the policeman, as evidence. He took the clothes to have them tested.

When the nurse suggested I call someone to have them bring me more clothes, I saw this as my chance. Instead of calling Steve, I called Julie and asked her to call Steve and tell him what had happened. I was afraid he might hang up on me in disgust, if I called. But I knew he wouldn't hang up on Julie.

"Tell him I swear I won't drink anymore, Julie. And this time I really mean it."

An hour or so later, Steve came by the hospital with my change of clothes. I was sitting on the exam table, crying, in a paper hospital robe. When I saw him, I reached out to him for a hug, hoping maybe he'd feel a little sorry for me. But he kept his distance. He handed me my bag of clean clothes, then pulled away with an empty look on his face. It was a look that said he'd totally given up on me.

"I brought you your clothes, Linda. But that's it," he told me. It looked like it was hard for him to say, but he'd already decided to say it. When Steve made a decision, he rarely changed his mind. "I can't be with an alcoholic. You don't even know what you're doing when you get drunk. You had sex with another guy. I can't believe it…"

"I know, Steve. You're right," I whimpered. "But I promise…"

"I'm breaking up with you, Linda. It's over."

As Steve said that last sentence, his lip quivered and tears came to his eyes. I hadn't ever seen him look so sad before. It scared me, because I'd never seen him look that way, so I believed him. The thought of losing Steve scared me. But the thought of being alone scared me even more.

Steve silently turned around, and slipped out the door. I started crying hysterically. I felt totally alone.

* * *

When I was finally released from the hospital, Julie picked me up and took me to get my car parked at Nadir's. I went home and took a shower, then crawled into bed. I felt so alone and depressed. The whole thing had turned into such a horrible ordeal. It was hard to comprehend how badly everything had gone.

Later that evening, the police called to tell me they were going to hold Nadir in jail for the next few days until I decided whether I would press charges. I thanked them and turned off the lights.

By Monday morning, I felt so drained that I called my boss Tom and told him I had some personal issues that came up and I wouldn't be at work for a few days.

In the afternoon, I got a call from the Rape Crisis Center. The counselor urged me to make Nadir stay in jail, if he really did rape me.

"You know, I don't know if Nadir raped me or not," I told her, honestly. "I don't remember what happened that night after I got drunk."

"He still shouldn't have had sex with you if he knew you were too drunk to know what you were doing," she said, reassuringly. "I say, keep him in jail a while longer. He deserves it."

A few minutes later Elizabeth called. Years before, Elizabeth had worked for Tom, my boss, and they'd stayed in touch. Apparently, Nadir had used his one phone call to call Tom because he didn't know anyone else in Santa Barbara and considered Tom a friend. Tom had called Elizabeth because he knew we were friends. He wanted to get as much information out of her as possible.

So by the time I called on Monday morning, Tom had already heard the whole thing from Elizabeth and Nadir. I wondered what he'd been thinking. He hadn't let on that he knew.

What was I going to do? Tom was not going to want me to work for him when I'd put his richest client in jail. "He's going to fire me," I told Elizabeth, before I hung up the phone.

Things were getting worse by the minute. I put my head in my hands and started crying. What a mess I was in. All because I'd had too much to drink one night. It was all so hard to fathom.

On Tuesday morning, a detective from the police department called me to say that if I didn't press charges, they'd have to let Nadir go. I had until the end of the day to call back with my decision. I called the Rape Crisis Center to ask what would happen if I pressed charges.

"Well, you'll be asked a lot of embarrassing and humiliating questions," she said. "But don't back down because of that. If you really believe you have been violated, you should press charges. It's the right thing to do."

I thought about it until I got the call from the police.

"You have to let us know now if you want to press charges," they said. "Otherwise, we have to let him go."

"I'm not pressing charges," I quietly told the policeman and Nadir was released.

* * *

When I went back into work, things were different. Normally, when I got to work each day, Tom would come out of his office, smiling, and say, "Good morning." We would always chat for a bit before getting down to work. It made for a friendly start to the day.

On Wednesday, Tom didn't come out at all. His door was closed. There was an envelope with my name on it sitting on my desk.

The letter inside was curt and to the point:

"Ms. Allan: According to the terms of your employment contract, you have been hired to work from 8:00 A.M. to 5:00 P.M., Monday through Friday. In the future, if you cannot be here during these agreed-upon hours, you must provide me with three days' notice. Failure to do so will result in immediate dismissal."

I called Elizabeth and read her the letter in a whisper, watching Tom's office door the whole time.

"I can't believe it," Elizabeth said.

"I'm going to quit," I told her.

"You HAVE to give two weeks' notice or you won't get a referral," she argued.

"Are you kidding? Tom isn't going to recommend me to anyone. No, I can't stand working here. I hate this job anyway. I don't even know how to do bookkeeping."

"Well, think about it for awhile before you do it," Elizabeth said, as we hung up.

I did think about it — for about two minutes. I had to quit — that day. I couldn't stand the humiliation of working there another minute with things the way they were.

Might as well do it sooner than later, I told myself. So I got up from my chair and walked into Tom's office. My legs were shaking.

"Tom, I'm giving you my notice," I said, as firmly as I could. Then I gulped hard and amended that. "Actually ... I'd like to leave today." I managed to get the words out.

"I think that's best," Tom said, with a relieved look on his face.

I really had nothing left to do before I walked out of the office for the last time, so I went back to my desk, looked things over, then happily walked out the door.

On the way home, I stopped by the supermarket. I was practically humming as I looked over the oranges and bananas. The guy who worked in the produce section noticed me smiling and said, "What are you so happy about?"

"I just quit my job," I said, ecstatically.

He started laughing. "I've never seen anyone so happy to quit their job."

* * *

I knew that if I didn't have Steve, my happiness over losing the job wouldn't last. I really wanted him back in my life. I didn't know what I was going to do, but I had to have him back.

A few days later, he gave me a little hope. In the middle of the afternoon, he called just to see how I was doing. I was excited to hear from him, but he made sure to keep the conversation short so I wouldn't think he might get back with me. I wanted to talk longer and tried to keep him on the phone, but Steve said he had to go and hung up. I was glad he'd called. I was starting to believe our break-up was temporary.

About a week after the incident, Steve called again. He reluctantly told me I could come over, just to talk. "But not to spend the night," he insisted.

A little smile came into my heart. I almost felt like giggling. I rushed over to his house on my best behavior. When Steve talked, I listened politely. He made a few gentle remarks about my behavior lately and I was careful to agree with him and look appropriately chastened.

As we sat on the couch and talked, I could sense that

Steve had been lonely and missing my touch. So I reached over and touched his arm, while we were talking, and gave him a warm, loving smile.

He smiled back.

That was what I'd been waiting for. Taking a chance, I stood up to hug him. Steve stepped into my arms.

"You were a bad girl," he said, quietly, holding me tight. "You're not going to do that again, are you?"

"No, Steve. Of course not," I promised.

We stood there holding one another for a long, long time. It was so good to be back in his arms.

"I love you, Steve," I said, blinking back the tears. "I'm so sorry I did this to you. It was horrible when I thought I might not ever see you again…"

And I ended up spending the night, after all.

21

I Quit

IF YOU'D ASKED ME, THE DAY BEFORE I QUIT, IF I'D EVER give up drinking, I'm sure I would have said, "No." I certainly wasn't planning on it. It happened in a single moment and I haven't wanted a drink since.

It was the night before my thirty-first birthday. Steve was planning to take me to dinner on Saturday, my birthday night, so I was celebrating with my family the night before. They were meeting me at my favorite restaurant at six thirty.

It was flattering to be remembered, but I didn't really enjoy these family birthday dinners. To my mom, they were an important family tradition, so we always got together. And it hadn't taken me long to discover that it really helped if I was buzzed. Sitting through a meal with the family didn't seem so boring.

Always willing to help out, Julie agreed to have our own little happy hour at the apartment and celebrate my birthday — just the two of us. She bought me a six-pack of beer and a pack of Eve menthol cigarettes for my birthday present. I laughed and thanked her for the "thoughtful" gifts. How well she knew my tastes.

It was literally an hour before we had to meet Mom, Craig and his fiancée Martha at the restaurant. So we drank fast. I guzzled three beers as quickly as I could, and Julie did away with most of a bottle of red wine before we left.

When we arrived at the restaurant, they were waiting in the parking lot. We all went in together.

"Five for dinner," I told the hostess. "But we'd like to have a few drinks at the bar first."

Mom frowned. "Wouldn't you rather have a drink at the table, once we've ordered?"

No, I really wouldn't. "Mom … it's MY birthday. I want to sit at the bar first." It had been almost thirty minutes since I'd had a beer and I was getting antsy.

Julie and I took our usual table in the corner. As soon as we sat down, a cocktail waitress we recognized came by. "One lite beer, one Chablis?" she said.

"Yes," Julie and I said, laughing.

"My mom and brother are here with us tonight celebrating my birthday," I told her. I was hoping she'd bring me a free beer, since I was a regular and I always tipped well, to guarantee good service.

The cocktail waitress left and when she returned with our drinks, she told me, "Your beer's on the house. Happy Birthday."

I finished the beer in about fifteen minutes and was ready for the next one. I knew Mom would give me a hard time if she saw me order another one that soon so I had to be discreet going about getting my next drink.

I excused myself from the table. "I'm going to the restroom," I said. On the way, I stopped to tell the bartender, "Could you send another lite beer to my table?"

I noticed how much the four beers had hit me. As I walked past the tables in the cocktail lounge I made eye contact with the people sitting at their tables, drinking. I felt so elated that I wanted to stop and talk to all of them — at least to say hi. I wished I could feel this way all the time.

A few minutes later, when I walked back to the table, I was excited to see from a distance that my new beer was waiting for me.

"Who ordered that beer?" Mom asked.

"I have no idea, but I'll take it," I said, grinning. By the time I'd finished my second beer in the bar, the hostess had come by to take us to our table for dinner.

Soon the waiter was pouring water for all of us and asking, "Would anyone like something from the bar?"

"I'll have a lite beer," I said, immediately.

"Why don't we not drink any more?" my mom said, diplomatically. "We can just look at the menu and order." She could see I was a little bit tipsy, but she had vastly underestimated my determination. I wanted my beer.

Imitating her sternness, I scowled in an exaggerated way, then leaned close to the waiter for a conspiratorial whisper. "I'll have a lite beer," I hissed.

My mom was not amused. "You've already had two beers. I think that's enough, don't you?"

Well, no. The answer to that ridiculous question was "NO."

"Mom, it's my birthday. You don't have to have any more, but I want to." I winked at the waiter and gave him a nod, letting him know the order was still on.

To my annoyance, he just stayed there, looking uncertain about whether to bring me my beer.

"Look," I said, making my point in a sarcastic tone. "It's my birthday… I want another beer. You're the waiter, aren't you? Why can't you just go and get the damn beer? It's okay."

Giving me a look, the waiter skulked away. Everyone at our table buried their faces in their menus, trying to ignore the tension. Eventually, the friendly cocktail waitress from the bar set a beer down in front of me. I drank it before the waiter came back for our orders.

"What can I get you?" he asked me, when he'd taken everybody else's order.

After six lite beers in about two and a half hours, I couldn't imagine eating. I wasn't hungry. I knew it wouldn't go over well, but I was too high to care. "I'm not hungry," I told him, closing the menu, decisively. "I'll take another beer though…"

Mom heard me. "No, Linda. You have to eat something."

"I'll eat bread. I'm not hungry, Mom."

"If you don't eat, we're all going to leave. We're not going to sit here and eat, while you just have a beer."

Mom and I started arguing, while Craig, Julie and Martha sat there watching us bicker. Nothing my mom said would've changed my mind. I was determined to have another drink. And I had the advantage. I knew my mom didn't like commotion. She was really invested in making everything nice when we got together. That's what these family birthdays were about. I waited for her to cave in. And she did.

"Okay. Have your drink," she said, grimly, after a few more futile attempts to change my mind.

The others ordered their dinners and ate, while I nursed my seventh beer.

As soon as I finished it, I was anxious to leave. There was no way I could order another drink in front of my family, so I started thinking about where I could go next. I could go home to drink in peace, but tonight was supposed to be my birthday celebration. Why not find some people to party with? There were a lot of bars downtown and I knew there was likely to be somebody I knew at any of them. But if I didn't know anybody, so much the better. I loved meeting new people when I was buzzed. I couldn't wait to leave, so I hurried things along.

Mom paid for the dinner and drinks, then we headed toward the parking lot. We got to my car first.

"Thank you, Mom," I said, giving her a peck on the cheek.

I rummaged around in my purse for my car keys, but couldn't seem to find them, so I twisted it around and searched harder. Somehow the purse slipped out of my hands and fell onto the asphalt, spilling the contents onto the ground. "There they are," I cried, happily, seeing the keys dumped out beside everything else. I bent over, unsteadily, to pick them up. Luckily, the car door was nearby. I leaned against it to keep my balance.

Mom stepped toward me and said, firmly, "Give me the keys. I don't think you should drive, Linda."

"I can drive. I'm not going far," I insisted. I unlocked the door, got into my car and closed the door right in front of her.

But Mom wasn't giving up. She knocked on my window and motioned for me to roll it down. I rolled it down partway. "I don't want you to drive. Let me take you home."

"Mom, I can drive. Don't worry about me."

Craig, Julie and Martha were standing at a distance, watching us. I thought for a moment they might be on my side, but apparently not.

"Linda, come on," Craig called out. "You can't drive like this. Do you want Martha and me to take you home?"

"Give me your keys, Linda. Come on, give them to me." Mom was persistent. "I won't let you drive when you're drunk."

I hated to admit she was right, but I was drunk and knew I shouldn't drive. All I really wanted was another drink. How was I going to get another drink, if I didn't drive?

Now Julie called out to me. "You can't drive, Linda." What nerve she had! She was my drinking partner. She'd been drinking drinks with me for the last three hours. Now she was telling me I couldn't drive? How could they all gang up on me like this? It was my birthday.

Craig, the most mellow, practical member of our family, walked over to me. "Come on, Linda, get out of the car," he said, calmly.

Reluctantly, I opened the door and Craig helped me out. "Listen, there's no reason for you to drive. One of us can take you, all right?" He didn't try to argue or make me feel like something was wrong with me. His voice was loving and concerned. Ever since David's death, Craig had been protective of Julie and me. If he was intervening, I knew he must've thought I was in danger.

As I leaned against the car, that idea started to sink in. What if I did get into an accident and die, like David? Or, even worse, what if I killed somebody else?

215

Two years before, Elizabeth had said something that had stuck in my mind. "Don't think it's not possible for you to crash into somebody when you're drunk. Maybe there's a woman who has a couple of kids at home and she's out running errands. You crash into her and kill her, so her kids don't have their mommy anymore. It could happen to you. It happens all the time."

Something in Elizabeth's voice that night had made me realize how wrong I'd been to believe it couldn't happen to me. What stupid thinking that was. Since that night, I'd never driven drunk again. So what was I doing now?

I gave my mom the keys.

It had been about twenty minutes since I'd had a beer. When I was as high as I was that night, I could feel my personality shift to anger if I couldn't continue drinking. The alcohol was wearing off and making me tense. I needed more beer to feel soothed and relaxed again. But I was going to have to lose these people pestering me first. I didn't know where my next drink would come from. I just knew I wasn't done drinking that night. Not by a long shot.

My mom got into the driver's seat of her car and asked me to get in too. I had a stick shift and she didn't like driving my car. She said she'd drive me to get my car the next morning. I felt trapped. If I let her take me home now, I definitely wouldn't be able to drink anymore. Even if I went with Julie, I knew she wouldn't stop by a liquor store either, because she was technically drunk and would insist on driving straight home. She had wine left from the day before at home anyway. I still had three beers at home, but that wouldn't be enough for the night. I couldn't see a way out.

And then I had what I thought was a brilliant idea.

"Wait a minute," I told my mom. "I have to go to the bathroom first. I'll be right back."

I started walking over to the restaurant. When I got close to the front door, I glanced back to make sure I was out of their view, then I cut across the street to a bar that Julie and I went to all the time. My shoulders relaxed as soon as I got inside the door. I'd escaped.

The bartender recognized me. "One lite beer?" she said. I nodded and she brought my beer right away.

I sat at the bar alone, drinking my beer and smoking a cigarette. A tingling feeling swept over me as I started to feel good again. A few more beers and things would be just fine.

Then my mom walked through the door.

It had only been about ten minutes. I couldn't believe she'd found me. I thought they'd wait a little while, then give up and go home. I wanted so much to drink alone.

Mom sat down next to me.

"What are you doing here?" I whined. "I want to be alone. Go home, Mom. I'll get a cab." I didn't like my mom to see me when I was drunk. And tonight, I had every intention of getting a lot drunker. She was spoiling my high.

The bartender came over. "A bottled water," my mom said.

Mom wasn't leaving.

"When we couldn't find you at the restaurant," she told me. "Julie said you might be here."

"Where's Julie?" I asked.

"Craig and Martha took her home."

"I don't want you here." I was feeling emotional and slurring my words. "Just go and leave me alone."

Mom's demeanor changed. She became direct. "No. I'm going to stay right here with you," she said, tapping her fingernail on the wood of the bar with a clicking noise. "All night, if I have to."

Her tone was firm, but I could see the pain in her eyes as she said it. Here I was, trying to drink myself into oblivion, and my mom was going to sit here next to me with bottled water, so she could be sure I'd get home safely. What had I done to deserve that kind of devotion? "I'm not a good daughter," I said and I started to cry.

"Yes, you are," she said, intently. "And I'm not going to leave you here alone."

Her eyes welled up with tears as she said those words to me. Even as drunk as I was, I could see how upset she was. And it startled me.

My mom was not the type of person to get tears in her eyes like that. In all my life, the only time I'd ever seen her get emotional was when David died. She'd cried a lot when she lost David. Did she think she was losing me now?

In that moment, something changed in me forever.

I knew my mom had already gone through the hell of losing her sixteen-year-old son because one of his buddies had been driving too fast. Now she was so worried about me that she was willing to sit here all night, watching me get drunker and drunker, if that's what I wanted. But the worried look in her eyes was unmistakable. She must have thought I'd be the next to die.

*   *   *

I wasn't in a party mood anymore. The drinks were paid for... My mom must have paid. I don't remember. But I wanted to go.

I sat glumly in the passenger seat while she drove me home. A hell of a birthday this was turning out to be. I was feeling sorry for myself, still floating in an alcoholic haze, when we came to a slow stop at an intersection. On the corner, I saw the gay bar where Steve's friend, Rick, used to sing. What a fun place that was.

Without warning, I jumped out of the car and stumbled toward it, leaving the car door open behind me. By the time I shoved open the swinging door, the memory of my mom in the car was ancient history. Here was a place I could get another drink and have some fun. I went right up to the bar and sat down.

The bartender's face darkened when he saw me, but he came over anyway.

"A lite beer," I slurred, happily.

"I've been ordered not to serve you if you came back in here again," he said, matter-of-factly.

He didn't offer any explanations, but I could see it would be futile to ask him again. So I just sat on the stool, dazed, trying hopelessly to clear my head. To this day, I don't know what I could've done to make them ban me from a gay bar.

My mom appeared and took my arm. "Let's go home."

On the ride home, I was sullen. My head was down, my eyes were closed. I didn't say a word. When we arrived, Mom came in and stayed for a few minutes, talking to Julie. I think she wanted to make sure I wouldn't leave again.

On her way out, she asked in a cheerful tone if I'd like to go to her club for lunch the next day, on my actual birthday. I said yes, then I went to bed and slept for twelve hours.

* * *

I woke up on my thirty-first birthday with a pounding headache. I kept going back to sleep, hoping that if I slept a little more the headache would subside. It didn't.

Finally, I got up around nine. Julie had left for work hours before, so I had the apartment to myself. I popped two Tylenol in my mouth while the coffee brewed, even though I knew it wouldn't help. Over the years, I'd found that nothing could take the miserable, pounding headache of a hangover away, except time.

I poured my coffee and walked back to my room. I felt sick. Why did I feel so lousy when I'd only had eight beers the night before? I felt like I'd had at least sixteen. There were the three with Julie, then the two at the bar, then … one, two … three after that. No, it was eight all right. So why did I feel like death?

Even the coffee tasted awful with the hangover. But I had to get caffeine in me or I wouldn't be able to function, so I forced it down.

I sat on my bed and turned the radio to my favorite rock-and-roll station, as I did every morning while I drank my coffee. In the mirror, several feet away, I could see myself, scowling, sitting on my bed and sipping coffee. I looked thinner because I was so dehydrated from all of the alcohol the night before. One good thing about drinking was that I always lost a few pounds after a night of drinking. But then, of course, I'd gain several pounds from drinking so much water the next day. Thinner on the day of the hangover, bloated the day afterward. That was my routine. Like listening to the radio, while I drank my coffee.

But somehow, that morning, the music bothered me. I wanted silence. I never had silence while I was drinking my coffee — I dreaded silence — but that day, I got up and turned off the radio. The silence was actually welcoming.

I threw my backrest against the back of my bed and sat down, curling my legs up next to me. I couldn't remember the last time I'd sat alone in my room, drinking coffee without my music blasting.

But this particular morning was different. I didn't fight the thoughts that came to me. In fact, I welcomed them.

One after another, the comments people had made to me over the years came rushing back into my mind: "Your drinking is out of control." "I think you might have a problem." "I'll bet you don't even remember what you did last night." "Haven't you had enough?"

Every one of these remarks had made me angry at the time. But after last night, they sounded different to me. It suddenly seemed so clear to me that these people weren't just trying to keep me from doing what I wanted to do. They were really worried about me. They'd said what they did because they cared. Why hadn't I seen that before?

Moments from dinner the night before flashed through my mind. It was as if I were standing on the outside, watching it all happen. There I was, drinking myself into a stupor, snapping at the waiter, arguing with my mom ... they'd all come out for my birthday and I'd ruined dinner for everyone. Not only had my mom seen me drunk, but I'd cried like a fool in front of her. I'd totally embarrassed myself. These people loved me. And all I'd been thinking about all night was how to get another drink.

My mom had literally sat next to me at that bar and given me unconditional love. I knew that even if I had sat at that bar, getting drunk all night, she would have sat there, right beside me, drinking bottled water, so she could drive me home. It was hard to ignore the power of that kind of love.

My dad says that unconditional love comes from God, that when my Mom showed me how powerful and absolute that love can be, it was really God working through her, because God is love.

I can't explain what happened that next morning. All I can say is that it felt like an epiphany. Suddenly I could picture myself living a life without alcohol. It was so clear to me in an instant. As I sat looking around my room, I thought, "What would a life without alcohol be like?"

For one thing, I'd never have to have another hangover again. I was having two to three hangovers a week and it was getting old. Although I didn't like to think about it, I knew the stories of my drinking were getting worse too. Not only had I been arrested twice and humiliated myself and my friends countless times, but lately I couldn't even remember what I'd done. When I drank, there were a lot of things I didn't remember the next day. I was usually so well lubricated that the memories seemed to slip right out of my mind.

Like it or not, I was always hearing stories about things I'd done when I was drunk. Sometimes the stories sounded like me. Other times, it was like hearing about a total stranger, so I couldn't imagine being where they said I'd been or doing what they said I'd done.

After awhile I started to feel a little skittish.

I'd go into a bar or restaurant, thinking I hadn't been there for weeks, and it would turn out I'd been there the night before. Not only that, but I'd pissed somebody off or made a complete fool of myself in some mysterious way. They still remembered, but I had no idea what had happened.

A waitress or a bartender would give me a funny look when I came in, but I wouldn't know why. Had I left without paying the bill? Had I passed out or thrown up on the floor? Had I insulted one of the customers? Maybe they were just surprised to see me back again so soon. Or they were having a bad day and it had nothing to do with me. How was I supposed to know?

I couldn't go around asking people, "Did I do anything …I don't know, embarrassing or weird last time you saw me?" So I had to guess and worry.

I was ruining my life behind my own back.

* * *

I thought of something the host of that Sunday radio show was always saying: "If we only knew how powerful we all were." That phrase came back to me now.

"If I only knew how powerful I was…" I said aloud, as if making a wish, "then I could give up alcohol for good."

But it was more than a wish. It was reality. I could do it. I really could give up alcohol. It seemed so clear. Of course, I could … ohmigod.

In that moment, it was like seeing a preview of my life. If I didn't take another drink, I could go to the gym and lose the rest of my weight. (I weighed 165 pounds that day and still had twenty pounds to go.) I could finish college. And most importantly, I could bring God back into my life.

For the past year or so, I'd felt closer to God at times, then I'd drink too much, get drunk and lose that feeling. I didn't want to pray to God when I felt sick with a hangover, so I'd put it off. But the hangovers were getting closer together and there wasn't much time for God in between. If I quit drinking altogether, alcohol couldn't get in the way of my spirituality anymore.

I don't know that I ever made a decision to stop drinking. Something just shifted. I'd never been so open before. The choices had never been so clear. As soon as I saw them, there was no question. My decision was made.

The words "The nightmare is over" came to me as if out of nowhere and those words stuck with me all day.

My head was still pounding, but all of a sudden being hung over and sick was okay, because I knew I'd never feel this way again.

"Now, there will be times in my life when I'll go to bars and be offered a drink," I told myself, thinking ahead. "It's no good to turn down the drink, but secretly want it. Or to watch other people drinking and wish I could be drinking too."

It's one thing to give up drinking — to make yourself resist it. It's completely a different thing to give up wanting it. That morning, I felt such grace. I saw myself as having a clean slate in life. It was as if I'd woken up that morning on a path at the top of a hill. I'd glanced behind me, for one quick second, to see the past twelve years of my drinking life, and then I'd turned and gone down the hill on the other side, never to go back to that way of life again.

In the past, I'd always assumed that I would have to figure out why I needed to drink, before I could stop drinking. But on that morning, I just stopped. I had a whole new life to look forward to. I didn't know what that would entail, but I was excited about it.

* * *

The phone rang about an hour later. "Happy Birthday to you…" Mom sang to me. "How do you feel this morning?"

"Not very good, but thanks for the birthday wish," I said.

"Do you remember we planned on lunch at the club today? You can change your mind if you want to, if you don't feel well," Mom said.

"I didn't forget. I do want to go to lunch today. Let's go around noon?"

"I'll pick you up at ten minutes to noon," Mom said.

"Sounds good."

I got a few birthday phone calls, took a shower and got ready to go out with Mom for lunch. I felt stiff and my head still hurt, but I knew the worst was almost over. This was the last time I'd ever feel this miserable again. Knowing that gave me an amazing feeling of lightness.

* * *

When we got to the club, the waiter came up to our table and said, "Would you like anything from the bar?" After the night before, it must have made my mom uneasy. It was like déjà vu.

Maybe I'll just have one more glass of wine, so I can remember this day, I thought, anxiously. It would be the last glass of wine of my life. Then I realized I'd already begun my life without alcohol that morning.

"Coffee with cream," I said. The anxious feelings disappeared. I felt strong and peaceful. This is how it will be from now on.

Mom and I talked a lot during lunch that day. Well, I did most of the talking. I told her that I had given up drinking for good, starting on my birthday. Years later, she told me that, as soon as she saw the look in my eyes, she knew I'd never drink again. She said there was something about the conviction I had that day that I'd never had before. It convinced her on the spot that I was through with drinking for good. She couldn't have been happier to hear it.

Both of us were so excited about the possibilities that not drinking opened up for me. We talked about how I was going to finish college. I already had a two-year degree from a city college, but I was going to go on for my bachelor's degree. I didn't know what I'd major in or what college I'd go to, I just knew I would become a college graduate. It had always been one of my goals. And now I could finally achieve it.

I was starting to realize how many goals I'd left unfinished, because of drinking. The year before, I'd joined the gym but had never gone once and my membership lapsed. I was going to start going regularly and lose the rest of my weight I wanted to lose. Now I could finish anything because alcohol wasn't going to get in my way anymore.

Even after we drove back to my apartment, my mom and I sat in the parking lot for hours, talking about my plans and dreams.

Steve took me to a French restaurant for my birthday. I felt lousy, but I looked nice by the time he picked me up. When we got to the restaurant, the waiter came by to take our drink orders. Steve got a shot of Jack Daniels and I said, "Just water, please."

When the waiter walked away I told Steve how I wasn't going to drink anymore. I told him of my goals and how excited I was. Steve beamed. "I hope you mean it. That would be the best news you could tell me, Linda."

We had a birthday toast to me: Steve's Jack Daniels and my glass of water.

* * *

The next morning I woke up feeling wonderful. I thought of what a great life I was going to have without booze.

It's surprising to me now, but somehow that morning, I fully believed that I would only experience good, happy situations for the rest of my life. Alcohol had brought me so much misery that I was certain I'd be happy all the time without it. And I did feel great for about three months. But then the challenges of daily life started to catch up with me and I wasn't used to dealing with them.

In the past, I hadn't given my life much thought. I'd focused only on drinking and pushed everything else aside. After I quit drinking, I instinctively knew I had to make changes in my life — so I could begin a new life, without alcohol. I didn't know at the time how hard it would be, but I welcomed it. I was happy just knowing I could at least have a life, now that alcohol was out of the picture.

And hard at it was, I knew I had to break up with Steve.

I loved him but I needed to sort myself out. I didn't know who I was or what I wanted. In some ways, not much had changed since the day I left the Ming Tree Motel and I wondered how I'd fill my time without any interests or hobbies. Without drinking, I still didn't know what I liked to do. I hadn't spent time alone in years. And now I had a lot of thinking over to do.

I didn't put it off. I told Steve right away what I was feeling. He didn't want to break up. And for someone who hadn't been able to stand being away from her guy for one day in the past, it was pretty amazing that I made the decision and stuck to it. But the same strength inside me that made me realize it was time to quit drinking was informing me about my relationship too. I just knew it had to end.

"But it isn't fair. I've been waiting for you to quit drinking for three years," Steve cried, when I told him. "Now you've finally quit drinking and you're leaving me?"

"It's not because of you," I tried to explain. "You're a great guy. It's just that I've been sleeping overnight here with you nearly every night and I don't know how to be alone. I still love you, but my mind has been pickled by alcohol for years. I just need time by myself for awhile. I feel it in my heart. It's what I have to do."

Painful as it was, I packed the clothes I kept at his place and took them back to my apartment. I knew I was doing the right thing, but it made me feel bad for Steve and lonely too.

To make things worse, since I was at home a lot more, Julie and I started having fights. She was used to having the apartment pretty much to herself and she liked it that way. Now I was there every night, but I wouldn't drink with her, so I wasn't any fun. We lived in a kind of truce, keeping to ourselves in different parts of the house — me, in my room, reading books, which I hadn't done in years; Julie in the living room, drinking and watching TV. We barely spoke to each other.

Would I have to give up seeing my boyfriend and living with my sister too? It seemed like a lot to bear suddenly, but I didn't want to come home every day after work to Julie drinking and watching TV all night. It wasn't a good environment for me anymore.

* * *

I knew Julie missed going out to the bars with me. I had taught Julie how to drink and smoke and we had done a lot of partying together over the years. So the tension was building living in the same apartment now.

In the past I hadn't cared much that the apartment wasn't clean and neat. With my act cleaned up, I wanted to live in cleaner surroundings. This clearly wasn't a high priority for Julie.

One evening I had been out with a friend and returned home to find Julie buzzed and eating Chinese take-out. She was in her bathrobe, watching TV. The ashtray was full of cigarette butts, and the apartment was smoky and filthy.

I looked at Julie with disgust and thought, here was a

young woman wasting her life drinking and smoking way too much, not eating healthy food and living in a pigsty. I came down hard on her.

"This place is filthy," I said, picking up the ashtray on the coffee table and emptying it into the trashcan.

Julie gave me an oh-you-think-you're-so-much-better-than-me look and slurred, "Oh, you think you're so special because you quit drinking."

"No, I don't. But all you've been doing is sitting around drinking, smoking and watching TV hour after hour, sitting in a filthy place. That's not a life."

"Oh, shut up and get out of here," Julie said. She stood up, nearly falling over on the couch.

"Are you going to start doing your share of cleaning this place?" I asked.

"No," she said defiantly, winking at me while she took a drink from her wine glass. I knew that look. It meant, I heard you, now shut up.

I was all riled up. "I want you to move out. I can't stand living with you," I screamed as I stomped toward my bedroom.

"You move. I like it dirty," Julie said, her tone sarcastic, as she moved over to the refrigerator to get some more wine.
I turned around and walked toward her in a threatening way. I pushed her.

Julie put her glass down and came after me yelling, "Don't you push me." Then she threatened to hit me. I ducked and she laughed. "Gotcha," she said.

I pushed her hard back onto the couch and continued walking to my room. Julie picked up her Chinese food in the small container and hurled it at me. It missed me, but got all over the wall.

"You clean that up," I shouted, slamming the door to my room.

The food on the wall and floor remained there for days. Neither one of us would give in and clean it. Finally I couldn't stand it any more and cleaned it up. Soon after that Julie told me she had found a place to move into with a couple friends. I was worried about what I was going to do — how I could afford a place of my own — but I knew it was the best thing. I had met a nice guy at the company I was working at, and he suggested we move into a two-bedroom, two-bath place together. Out of fear, I moved in with Mark. It turned out to be a bad decision. We dated for several months before realizing we had nothing in common, except that we had both quit drinking.

Some people who give up drinking find it hard to be around other people who drink. They feel tempted to drink themselves. But for me, when I gave up drinking, I gave it up completely. I really didn't want it anymore. So it wasn't that I was tempted. I just didn't fit into a drinking environment. I didn't think I was better than Julie or anything. I just wanted something else. I knew that as soon as I could work out the logistics, I'd have to move.

Plus I couldn't believe how difficult my life was becoming. Without alcohol to help me ignore the tough times, I had to face them head on and it seemed like it would never end. I didn't understand what was happening. Instead of being happy, I was lonely and miserable. I found myself crying several times a week, just to relieve the pressure. Was this what it was like to live without alcohol?

* * *

Alcoholics are very self-centered people. When I drank I'd gotten into the habit of only looking out for myself. I don't think I ever truly saw who any of my friends or boyfriends really were. I didn't give them the chance. It was all about me. What could they do for me? How could they make me happy?

It took awhile to realize that all the time I was trying to find happiness in other people, I never felt happy. I was only distracting myself from how bad I really felt. That's avoidance, not happiness.

For some of us, finding happiness in ourselves does not come easily. It takes time and effort to find something deep inside that's valuable enough to make life worth living. Every moment you avoid it — by drinking or smoking or overeating, like I did — is a moment wasted. A moment you could've found happiness.

I drank for twelve years — from the time I was nineteen to thirty-one. I wasted some of the most important years of my life. Instead of facing my fears and going for the things I wanted in my life, I drank. When I think back on it now, I can hardly believe it. It wasn't easy to get my bearings after I gave up drinking. But I wouldn't spend one day living like that now.

* * *

For a long time, after I quit drinking, my weight stayed at 155. It was only about ten pounds higher than my ideal weight and, although I still wanted to get down to 145, I was working out, so my body was toned. I felt healthy and full of energy. Men noticed how I looked and gave me a lot of attention, which I loved.

One day, Gary, a salesman at the company where I was working, asked me out for drinks and dinner. I'd always enjoyed talking to him whenever he came in, so I told him I'd love to go.

The day before our date, I went shopping. Gary was a bright, engaging guy, definitely not one of the disappointing "safe dates" I'd looked for when I was fat. Why not make this date a special treat?

First, I tried on a soft, flowing, knee-length blue dress that I'd seen in the store window. It had long sleeves, with openings cut at the shoulder to reveal my arms and a tiny belt at the waist. I liked it. But it didn't really excite me.

I left the dressing room and wandered back out to the dress department. Most of the dresses were fine, but I wanted something special. A seductive, white angora top caught my eye. I could pair it with a clinging jersey skirt or even that purple number with the long slit up the thigh.

But just as I was turning to go try them on, my eyes drifted up. Across the room, on a display that led into the evening wear department was a little black dress. Not just any little black dress, a Little Black Dress, with every bit of magic that term can conjure.

Sexy, snazzy, off-the-shoulders cute and irresistible. THAT was the dress for me. It was definitely NOT the kind of dress you could wear if you were fat. "Short and sexy" always translates into "hideously embarrassing" if you look like a blimp. No amount of pretending you were actually thin would help. To make a hot little number like this work, you had to be thin. Or else. In fact, you pretty much had to look good naked or it wouldn't work.

So this was the moment of truth. There was no question that I had definitely lost a lot of weight — fifty five pounds, from my peak at 210. But did I look good now or did I just look "better"?

As if in a trance, I hung the skirts back on their racks and crossed the room to get closer to that dress. If it was on the mannequin, a whole assortment of sizes must be waiting nearby. I scanned the area. There they were, four little black dresses in a row, hanging quietly from a rack, as if they were just ordinary dresses.

I walked over to them and checked each one for size. Size 12. No. (Thank God!) Size 4. No. Size 4. Uh-oh ... Size 10. I breathed a little sigh and pulled the dress out, sizing it up at a glance to see if it looked like it would fit.

I hadn't quite locked in an accurate body image yet. Sometimes I still felt like I might end up in fat clothes, even when that was totally wrong. But I glanced at the mirror and glanced again at the dress and thought it just might work. I couldn't wait to try it on.

Once in the dressing room, I quickly got undressed. There was a time when I had faced the three full-length mirrors of these dressing rooms with trepidation. If I had to go in, I'd leave as many clothes on as possible and get out as quickly as I could, so I wouldn't have to stand face-to-face with myself in bad lighting and realize I looked fat from any angle.

Those days were gone. I pulled off my top and quickly dropped my jeans to the floor. The lighting in the room still sucked, but hey, I looked pretty damn good anyway. And I wanted to see myself in all three mirrors — to make sure I looked great from all sides. What a turnaround.

I took the little black dress off the hanger and pulled it over my head. It slid down my body effortlessly, caressing all the right curves. The fabric was light and moved with my body. I couldn't help but swish my hips and smile.

I looked like one of those girls on TV who used to make me think, "What on earth does she eat? I don't think I'll ever be that thin."

And now I was that thin.

* * *

Gary had always seen me at work, looking my best, but in a workaday style that didn't really offer much pizzazz. When I opened the door the night of our date, he smiled and his smile just kept getting bigger as he looked me over.

The thin me was a hit.

That night, I laughed more than I ever had with a man. We talked all the way to the El Encanto Hotel, where we were to have dinner. When we parked, Gary came around and opened the door for me. He put his arm out, so I could hold onto him, as we walked into the restaurant, talking and laughing.

As soon as we sat down in the bar, the cocktail waitress

came over to take our drink orders.

"Bottled water for me," I said.

"Bottled water?" Gary said, curiously.

"Sparkling water or plain?" the waitress asked.

"Just plain."

Gary smiled. "Are you sure?"

"Yes. I don't drink."

"Bring me a bottled water too," he said to the waitress. "I don't drink either."

When the waitress left, I explained to Gary that I'd "had" to quit drinking several years before. We were getting along so well, I was really hoping he'd understand.

"Are you an alcoholic?"

"Yes, but I don't usually say that. It's just that I can't drink anymore."

He explained that he was an alcoholic too and had quit drinking fairly recently. We sat and talked over our bottled waters for about an hour, then I asked him if he minded if I stepped outside to have a cigarette. At that point, I was down to four a day and I really wanted one before dinner.

"Oh, I'm so glad you said that," he exclaimed. "I've been DYING for a cigarette."

We laughed and went out to the patio to have our cigarettes. I led the way and smiled quietly to myself, realizing that I didn't mind at all that he was following behind me, watching the swish of my dress. I looked great from behind.

For that matter, I looked great from the left and from the right as well. That dressing room mirror had revealed it all. I looked fine. And it was about time.

Gary and I had a wonderful dinner and great conversation the rest of our date. When he dropped me off at home, I thanked him for the really nice evening and gave him a quick kiss and went inside.

I never dated him again, but as I walked into the house and shut the door behind me, I knew that this was the kind of date I'd always wanted to go on — a date with an appropriate man who found me attractive, treated me well and gave me lots of attention, a date where weight was not an issue and drinking was not an issue.

I felt proud of myself for having come as far as I had. Giving up drinking and losing fifty-five pounds were accomplishments in their own right, even if I had a little further to go. And this night, the Night of the Little Black Dress was my first real proof that I had a great life waiting for me up ahead.

* * *

Smoking was a different story. Whenever I'd start to contemplate a life without cigarettes, I wouldn't allow myself to finish the thought. It was difficult even thinking about it. I knew my attachment to them was more emotional than physical. But I just HAD to have my two cigarettes per day.

People would ask me, "Why don't you just quit, if you're only smoking two a day?"

And I'd think, "Because I WANT my two cigarettes a day. It's my treat. It's my special time all alone, smoking and thinking things over. I look forward to it. I LOVE my two cigarettes! I can't give that up — I WON'T!"

And then I got sick.

In the middle of January 2001, I had one of the worst colds in my life. It was one of those colds that seem to take over your body. Your head throbs, your sinuses are clogged. If you try to speak, your voice is unrecognizable. If you try to eat, you can't tell the difference between hot Szechwan and creamy Italian, because you can't taste a thing.

I took as many cold pills as I dared, but it barely phased the cold. For a week or so, it was all I could do to drag myself out of bed every day and get to work.

The thing is, with this nasty cold, smoking wasn't

enjoyable at all. The smoke tasted awful. And my lungs were fighting it. They were so filled with congestion already, there was really nowhere for the smoke to go. I knew smoking would only make my cold worse. Like it or not, I was going to have to give it up for the next few days. I wasn't looking forward to that.

After about four days not smoking I was feeling irritable. I'd had a particularly rough day at work and promised myself a cigarette when I got home. I was still coughing and congested with the cold, but four days was enough. Whether it tasted bad or not, I was going to smoke a cigarette.

As soon as I made the decision, I started to smile. I looked forward to that cigarette for hours. The rest of the day might be going to hell, but I was going to make one thing go right for sure.

By the time I left work and drove home, I was in a bad mood. My only solace was that cigarette I'd be having when I got home. I walked into my house and instead of feeding my two hungry cats, I threw my things on the bed, grabbed a cigarette and lighter and went outside to smoke. The cats looked offended. They were getting used to being fed the minute I got home. But they'd have to wait. I was so looking forward to this — and I deserved it. This would be a sweet experience.

I lit the cigarette and took a puff. The taste was horrible. It reminded me of the first time I smoked and how ghastly the taste of the cigarette was then. I quickly took a second puff, hoping the regular taste — the taste I loved so much and had been missing all week — would return. It didn't.

Now it was my turn to be offended. I looked at the cigarette like my cats had looked at me. How could it betray me like this? I'd been looking forward to this cigarette for hours!

I tried again. The third puff not only tasted awful, it also made me feel a bit light-headed. I took a deep breath to try to get rid of the wooziness. Then I took another puff. The fourth one was the worst. I not only felt faint, but my stomach quickly went sour, as if I were going to throw up. I knew I couldn't smoke any more that night.

I reluctantly put my cigarette into my little ashtray I kept outside for my two cigarettes a day. The ashtray was filled with water from the heavy rains the night before.

Before I dropped the cigarette into the ashtray, I looked at the cigarette. I'd only smoked about half of it. Should I try one more puff? No. Not tonight. I hated the nauseous feeling and was afraid of literally getting sick. As I dropped my half-smoked cigarette into the ashtray, I wondered, Could this be the last cigarette I'd ever smoke? Has the time finally come?

I stopped the thought. I wouldn't be smoking anymore today — just today. I made a specific point not to project anything about the future.

* * *

The next day was Saturday. After spending the afternoon enjoying the park down by the beach, I came home and cleaned up the house a bit. I'd also started taking singing lessons. Around four o'clock I thought, "It's time to smoke…" But I just picked up my sheet music, put my tape in my cassette player and practiced my singing instead.

This turned out to be a cleverer ruse than I'd expected. Since I usually didn't practice my singing lesson until after I'd had a cigarette, singing made me think I'd already had my cigarette!

When I was getting ready for bed that night, I was aware of the time when I would normally go outside and smoke. Instead, I turned down my bed and crawled under the sheets. I still felt noticeably mellow and upbeat and didn't allow myself to think too deeply about not having my usual cigarette. I slept well that night.

This routine worked so well that I kept it up for the next several days. Any time I caught myself thinking. What about your cigarettes? or Don't you miss your cigarettes? or Are you quitting? I pictured the thought sort of stopping in mid-air, never finishing. I wouldn't respond to the question, I'd just let it stop and wait there, while I moved my mind into a calm, relaxed place instead.

The Tibetan monks who have been quieting their thoughts in meditation for thousands of years say that it does no good to try to resist your thoughts and push them out of your head. It's much more effective to accept them and ignore them. Just let them float by. Don't give them any energy. And that's what I did. It was incredibly helpful in allowing me to quit smoking.

Gradually, I began to see that when thoughts about smoking came up, they didn't affect me anymore. I was more surprised than anyone to find myself a non-smoker. But I knew I was finally free from cigarettes. And it was a good feeling.

That day after I became sick smoking the half cigarette turned out to be the first day I quit smoking, but I didn't know it at the time. I felt so light and relaxed all day. But months later, when I looked back to those several days when I initially quit, I remembered that feeling of lightness. It was a sense of God's presence that I have felt many times before. I really believe that God just gave me that little boost I needed in the beginning so that I could once and for all drop my smoking habit.

I also think that it was just time for me to quit. After twenty-eight years of "fun," it was time to get a deeper sense of God. I had lost my weight, quit drinking and now quit smoking. So there was nothing to get in between God and me. I think that's why I got the help. I never asked for help to quit smoking, but I surely needed it.

It's great to not be beholden to cigarettes anymore. It didn't happen immediately, but over time as the thoughts and memories about smoking dissipated, there finally came a point when I knew I was free.

22

Looking Back

W HEN I WAS FAT, MY WHOLE WORLD REVOLVED AROUND being fat. And when I was drinking, my whole world revolved around getting my next drink.

Whether I got my sugar high from candy bars or Chips Ahoy or Miller Lite, I was just reaching out for that sweet moment of euphoria. It was always fleeting. But it was all I knew of happiness.

I didn't understand that happiness cannot be found in a self-centered life. And addicts are, by nature, self-centered. I was living in a state of panic. Drinking, smoking and eating were my ways of coping with my fears. I had so many fears and instead of looking for solutions, I took the easy way out, every chance I could get.

There's nothing anyone could do about my drinking until I wanted to stop. Everyone close to me made comments about how much I drank. My family, friends and boyfriends all told me I had a problem with alcohol. For the first ten years or so, I didn't think I had a drinking problem. I just saw myself as drinking a little too much sometimes.

Even when I did accept the fact that my drinking was a problem, no one could make me quit. On the day I quit, I was the one who made the decision. Nobody else. It just wasn't going to happen until I decided to do it, no matter what anyone said to me.

Looking back now, I see how many men's hearts I broke. During the years I drank, I had a lot of boyfriends and I hurt every one of them with my drinking. At the time, I didn't care if I hurt them. In the end, I had missed out on finding a man I could fall in love with and possibly marry.

All the women's groups kept saying women didn't need men and I believed them. I decided I would live with men and have sex with men, but I would make it on my own. Now, I didn't realize that I was eating and drinking away my best years for making a life with someone and having kids. So I missed out.

I can still fall in love with someone, of course. I'm not dead yet. And with or without a man, I can certainly adopt kids. I probably will. But nothing I can do will turn my biological clock back, so I can have kids of my own. Nothing will give me back those lost years.

* * *

When I was fat, I wasn't really living. It was as if my life was on hold. I was too fat to be the person I knew myself to be inside. So I constantly had thoughts about "the other life" I'd live when I lost the weight. In that life, I could be happy.

I'd see commercials on TV with beautiful girls in bathing suits at the beach, laughing and running in the sand without any self-consciousness at all. They didn't have to pull their skirts down awkwardly to cover their fat legs or wear jackets over everything to hide their big bellies and create a "smooth silhouette." They'd throw off their clothes and strip down to bikinis and still look good from every angle. I could only imagine what that would be like.

I knew I had it in me. Deep inside, I could feel that I was the kind of person who could be happy in my body. It was easy for me to see myself, thin and confident, going out into a crowd of strangers with perfect ease. I knew that, if I could only be myself, people would like me and accept me. And I could feel great about my life too.

But one look in the mirror could sap my confidence.

When I was fat, I didn't feel like me. I couldn't talk to people or try new things or be happy with my personality. I was overcome with self-loathing. As a fat person, I spent a lot of time mad and depressed. I shut myself off from the world and spent my time hating my body and my life.

Today, when I see people on TV insisting they are fat and happy, I don't believe it for a minute. I think they've just given up and are trying to make the best of a bad situation. In our society, fat people will always be looked down upon as being lazy and having no discipline. It doesn't matter how much fat people try to explain that they are not lazy and undisciplined, the stigma lingers. Even if the medical researchers finally manage to prove that some fat people are fat because of their genes, it won't help. The lumpy, flabby, unappealing nature of fat will still put people off — whether it's on their own body or somebody else's. We may not all want to be as thin as a supermodel, but we all want to look good and be fit. It's human nature.

In my case, I know I wouldn't have cared nearly as much about my life or future if I had stayed fat. When I didn't care about my body, I didn't care about my life that much either. I was coasting. The pressure of trying something new or taking up an ambition made me turn to food and hide.

Sometimes I think about how my life would have been if I hadn't lost weight. I don't think I would have gone on to finish college. I would never have gone to the gym, which I now love. I wouldn't have been as open to relationships or new friends. And I would definitely not have had the confidence I do now. Now that I'm thin, it's easier to relax and be myself, because I feel like the person I truly am.

For all of those years, I was compulsively eating to steal a moment of happiness from life, as if that was the best I could do. When actually, the thing that's made me happier is not eating compulsively. Eating healthy food and working out have given me the thin, toned body I always dreamed of. In this body,

I feel happier when I'm sitting in a chair, doing nothing, than I ever did stuffing cookies into my mouth.

* * *

I always associated alcohol with happiness too. But the truth is, it didn't bring me happiness at all. It kept me from living a full life. I used alcohol to avoid having to do things. I wasted a lot of time drinking, frittering my life away.

The day I quit, I told myself I was going to give up alcohol for good. And I have.

I'm perfectly content to drink water or juice whenever I go out. People drink around me and it doesn't bother me. I don't feel like they're putting me in the path of temptation. It's my responsibility not to drink, not theirs. I never put myself in situations where people are drunk, because being around drunken people just isn't any fun, if you're not drunk yourself, but I do go out to places where people drink.

I have such a freedom now because I don't have to drink. I used to live for the next drink and now it never crosses my mind. It's been so long since I did drink that it's almost as if I can't remember drinking at all. I haven't taken one sip of alcohol in twenty years and I really don't want it anymore.

* * *

At the same time, I have a more personal experience of God now. In the beginning, I tried to live a life with God in a private way. I didn't talk about God with anyone except my dad or Elizabeth. She had always seen me as a searcher and sensed God's importance to me. But I didn't realize how important it was to share ideas with other people and learn from their experiences.

But I quickly found that that way of life was too lonely, so I decided to open myself up to the possibility of going to churches or spiritual meetings of some sort. One day, I was out having coffee and started talking to a man in the coffee shop who was the host of a local, spiritual TV show. He invited me to his meditation group at his house and told me he would teach me how to meditate. When I went, I found it to be a good step toward developing my own spirituality and I met some interesting people there as well.

I go to different churches so I can meet people. One of my favorite things is to be there when the entire congregation is praying. I love that. In that moment, it feels as if I'm part of something so sacred. We're connecting with God. I'm always humbled by it.

Of course, I still have a lot of questions about God: Why does He seem to help some people and not others? Why is it so difficult to feel God at times? What is God, really? Will we know who God is when we die?

But in the silence — when I've prayed or meditated and felt touched by God's spirit — I feel so calm and reassured that it's easier to believe, and the questions don't seem to matter as much.

* * *

They say you need to replace an addiction with something else. For me, that something else is spirituality or God. My addictions to food, alcohol and cigarettes have been replaced by God. I think this is so important.

Whatever it was that made me feel I needed the addictions before, gradually dissolved over the years, when I replaced each addiction with God.

There was something now bigger than just my addictions and me. As my dad once told me, it's so much better than living my own small life. With my sense of who God is, I know I will never drink alcohol, smoke cigarettes or be fat again. I'm absolutely certain.

After I quit drinking, my dad often reminded me of his conviction that, without God, he didn't think anyone could completely give up an addiction. And I strongly agree.

My life is proof that addictions can be given up for good. I'm not fighting off my addictions. I am free. I don't have to try to prevent myself every day from eating junk. I don't go out for a dinner and watch everyone around me drinking and wish I could have a beer. I don't turn my head away and think, "I really want a beer, but I can't ever have that again!" It's done. It's over.

It's the same with cigarettes. The smell of cigarettes can be incredible. I have to admit: I do still love the smell of cigarettes, except early in the morning. Yuck. But I don't want to smoke cigarettes anymore. I can smell someone's cigarette and think, "That sure smells good," but I never even entertain the idea of smoking again. For twenty-eight years I was chained to cigarettes. There's nothing appealing about that to me any more. Whether it smells good or not, I have no desire to smoke again.

I have that experience with food now too. When I pass the vanilla ice cream at the supermarket or see someone up ahead of me in line with a big bag of chocolate chips, I have to smile. They sure taste good. I can't help but remember that. But if I take a glance at my reflection in the window, as I leave the store, or notice how healthy I feel, I know there's no way that I'd trade any amount of sugar for that!

And the rewards of giving up addictions are even greater. By the time I'd gotten to a weight I was comfortable with, I had already given up smoking and quit drinking too. With each accomplishment, I feel more confident about taking bigger risks, so my life keeps getting better and better!

Writing this book is a perfect example. I thought about writing this book three years ago, then my mother's husband died, then one of my ex-boyfriends died. After each one of these deaths, I didn't think about the book for months. But I didn't forget about it either. I knew I was going to have it published, one way or another. I didn't know how, exactly, but I knew it would become a reality. And here it is.

As I tackle each new challenge, it's finally starting to sink in: I can really do just about anything I set out to do. Knowing it is one thing. Proving it again and again in my own life is even better. Every time I do something hard and succeed, it just makes me bolder the next time.

I can't wait to see what happens next.

Epilogue

LIFE WAS NOT THE BED OF ROSES THAT I THOUGHT IT WAS going to be after giving up my struggle with addiction.

I knew better, of course. Life is challenging for the best of us. But I have to admit, I secretly thought that I had paid my dues and life would cut me some slack.

Instead, the next thing that happened was I fell for an alcoholic who smoked two packs a day and wouldn't dream of exercising or eating right. I don't mean we "dated." He was one of the loves of my life.

All of the emotions I had managed to avoid by putting candy bars or cigarettes or alcohol in my mouth came flooding over me with a vengeance. When people say I'm strong for being able to give up my addictions, I think of all the days I found myself crying, for apparently no reason at all, after I'd quit.

Over the years, most people develop a kind of resilience against the everyday pains and slights of life. But when you've avoided that pain by turning to addictions instead, you aren't used to facing life without a buffer. And let me tell you, it can be pretty terrifying.

Reality hit me hard. Without anything left to hide behind, I had to learn new skills for coping fast. But that's the next book, when the story goes on.

The main thing I want to say is that, no matter how hard life gets, facing life is infinitely better than trying to hide from life in an addiction.

I don't mean because it's "the right thing to do" or

"you'll be a better person for it." I mean because it's easier. Living as an addict of any kind is hard. Too hard. Much harder than being free.

I couldn't live one day like that again. And I never will.